OUTDOOR ADVENTURE FOR HANDICAPPED PEOPLE

HUMAN HORIZONS SERIES

OUTDOOR ADVENTURE FOR HANDICAPPED PEOPLE

by

Mike Cotton

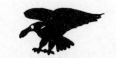

A CONDOR BOOK
SOUVENIR PRESS (E & A) LTD

First published 1983 by Souvenir Press
(Educational & Academic) Ltd,
43 Great Russell Street, London WC1B 3PA
and simultaneously in Canada

ISBN 0 285 64973 6 casebound
ISBN 0 285 64978 7 paperback

Photoset and printed in Great Britain by
Photobooks (Bristol) Ltd.

Acknowledgements

For eight years I was fortunate to be employed developing courses in outdoor leisure and education as warden of Churchtown Farm Field Studies Centre, in Cornwall. The environmental aspects of our work were described in my earlier book in this series, but equally important has been the experience we have gained in the organisation of courses in a wide range of adventure activities.

In writing this book I have been fortunate in having the assistance of all the staff at Churchtown Farm, who over the years have given me so much support in developing and teaching our courses. Further assistance has been given by friends and colleagues working in the field of leisure and recreational activities for mentally and physically handicapped people. These contributors have been able to give the expert and technical advice, all obtained at first-hand, which was desirable and necessary for the writing of certain chapters. In particular I should like to thank John Walker, a tutor in outdoor pursuits at Churchtown Farm, who wrote the chapters on sailing and rock-climbing; Len Warren, National Co-ordinator for Water Sports, British Sports Association for the Disabled, who has contributed the chapter on angling; Daphne Pagnamenta, a council member of the Riding for the Disabled Association, for her chapter on riding; and Fiona Freddi, an active committee member of the Uphill Ski Club, who wrote the final chapter on winter sports.

In addition I have received shorter sections from other contributors: David Owens, on cruise holidays; Jonathan Chapman, on the canoe expedition; and Dick Endres, on his excellent programme of winter activities at Camp Confidence, Minnesota. Others have supplied information and helped in many ways: Martin Lazell, Deputy Warden at Churchtown Farm; Ron Moore, (canoeing); Nigel Summerling (caving); Lynda Williams of the British Ski Club for the Disabled and members of the Uphill Ski Club (winter sports).

Illustrations have been provided by Sue Leake, who also did most of the art work for my previous book. She has been assisted by John Walker who has illustrated his own chapters. The photographs were mainly taken by David Owens and myself; others have been supplied by Beaumont College (swimming), Riding for the Disabled, Uphill Ski Club and by staff of summer camps in America which I visited in 1982 on a Winston Churchill Travel Fellowship. These were Bradford Woods Outdoor Education Center, Indiana; Camp Confidence and Camp Courage, Minnesota; Camp Elliott, Pennsylvania and Camp Wawbeck, Wisconsin.

Once again the typing and checking of the manuscript has been the responsibility of my wife, Sue, who has also accompanied, and shared with me, many of the adventures described in both books.

Finally, I should like to thank the Spastics Society, who had the vision to establish Churchtown Farm in 1974 and thus to give a taste of adventure and opportunities for leisure to so many handicapped people. In eight years there have been thousands of participants, young and old, mentally retarded and physically disabled, who have experienced with us the thrills of climbing and canoeing, hiking and orienteering, camping and sailing. To all of them this book is dedicated. I hope they enjoy reading of their exploits.

Contents

Preface

Leisure and recreation is of considerable importance to anyone concerned with the lives of handicapped people, and many who are disabled themselves have asked the question, 'Why cannot I participate alongside others?' Meaningful leisure has perforce become for many a substitute for meaningful employment, and while twenty years ago we were concerned with vocational training courses and sheltered employment, today we are more used to providing social and leisure education for those who are mentally retarded or physically disabled.

In hospitals, residential establishments, training centres and special schools and colleges, we find staff employed with the specific responsibility for developing and organising sport and recreation.

Clubs which formerly were merely meeting places for social functions are now looking to extend their activities out of doors and at the same time to develop integration with able-bodied youngsters.

The holiday scene, too, is rapidly changing to accommodate those handicapped individuals who are no longer satisfied with the traditional week at the seaside, with its dearth of recreational opportunities. Organisations concerned with disability have looked at this exciting demand by the population they serve and there has been a wide expansion of active holidays. Why not try sailing and canoeing? Go fishing by the banks of a Scottish loch? Take a winter holiday in Austria, Italy or Switzerland – and learn to ski among the snow and mountains? The world has suddenly become your oyster, even if you are disabled.

At the same time national sporting bodies have opened their doors to this rapidly expanding market, establishing separate organisations and committees to look at facilities, resources and programmes. The British Sports Association for the Disabled; the Advisory Panel on Water Sports for the Disabled; The British Ski Club for the Disabled; the Committee for Promotion of Angling for the Disabled . . . the list is almost endless.

Local recreation centres are keen to see handicapped people participating, either alongside others who are more able or during specific sessions arranged especially for them. Other centres have been built to cater for the demand, introducing mentally and physically handicapped people to new experiences by means of short courses in a residential setting. Often this can be the best way to try your hand at a variety of adventure activities with qualified, experienced staff present to meet your needs and give support when required. From there you can move easily out to the local clubs with at least the knowledge that you enjoy and can cope with a particular activity.

During the International Year of Disabled People, in 1981, there was great public awareness of the needs of disabled people – not least in the field of outdoor education and adventure activities. Many conferences and seminars brought people together – disabled and able-bodied – to discuss these needs. At one such national meeting I felt almost out of place alongside three disabled speakers, all of whom had not only contributed significantly to the development of sports and adventure pursuits for people with similar disabilities but had also achieved great personal satisfaction from active participation.

That year saw the appearance of several much needed books providing information on leisure and recreation, outdoor pursuits and specific activities for handicapped people. One such publication was my earlier book, *Out of Doors with Handicapped People*, to which the present work forms a companion volume. The first looked at environmental education in a practical way and formed a basis for the excitement of adventure education in this book. We examined the world of water, both in rivers, lakes and the sea. Now we can learn how to use those environments for pleasure and adventure – sailing, canoeing, cruising and fishing. We explored the high mountains and moorlands, looking at landscape, geology and wildlife.

How much more does this give to the rambler or backpacker walking the hills and feeling the excitement of wild country? The orienteer or expeditioner will always need knowledge of the climate and terrain, and an understanding of his environment may even aid his survival.

This book, it is hoped, will stimulate an interest in adventure out of doors for those with significant handicaps, and also for those who work with handicapped people. Whether you swim, sail or ski; climb, cave or canoe; or just wish that you could – this book will give you encouragement and we hope lead on to even greater adventure.

Introduction

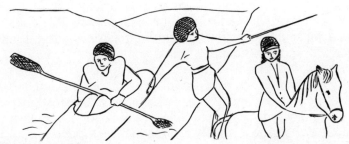

Why be active?

Ability or disability? How we approach the concept of *activity* depends largely on how we view the idea of handicap. Are the limitations too severe to contemplate much activity? Is there too high a risk factor? Is it easier to remain quiet and not be active? The list of questions we can pose is seemingly endless.

Often, where we stand on that issue will depend on 'which hat we are wearing' at the time – which viewpoint we adopt. The medical consultant, physiotherapist, recreation officer, teacher, parent . . . all will express differing opinions. But what of the handicapped persons themselves? Is it sufficient to have to remain always on the sidelines; watching activity from the outside; never being allowed to participate? How much better if we can try something for ourselves; not always succeeding, perhaps not always enjoying, but at least being actively involved. The days of mere observation are rapidly disappearing and horizons are expanding. The world of disability now seeks to merge more thoroughly into the world of ability; the handicapped person in society is not content to remain a spectator but is looking for the opportunity to participate. All those concerned with leisure and recreation should be opening their doors to meet this demand at every level.

But, why be active? Perhaps it is purely striving for normality. The mountain is there, so let's climb it; the sea is there, so let's cross it. Man has always sought adventure and striven to achieve the impossible – so why not the handicapped person? What makes the blind or deaf man, the paraplegic or amputee, the epileptic or haemophiliac, so very different from everyone else? *Really the difference is only in degree of ability –*

and at that point we are being positive. I personally know of a blind person who can ski much better than many who can see; of a paraplegic who can coach others, supposedly able-bodied, to sail; of an amputee who climbs mountains most people only hear of from books and television; and of many thousands of others who just want to 'have a go'.

We realise that activity is good for both body and mind – the active person is a happy person. Exercise, however strenuous or however simple, aids breathing and circulation, muscles and joints. The person normally confined to the wheelchair may be released from its limitations on entering water in the pool or on lying horizontally on a floor mat in the gymnasium. Freedom of movement, exercise, will make the remainder of the day seem so much better when one is once again seated in that same chair. Many activities will help relaxation, both of muscles and mind. Swimming and yoga are well known therapies which apply equally well to the able and to the disabled. But what about the therapeutic value of fishing or sailing, rambling or skiing? Outdoor activities can be just as beneficial to body and mind. We simply need to expand our attitudes, widen our horizons and give an opportunity to *everyone* to join in.

Adventure – an idea for handicapped people
Adventure can vary as much as do individuals and what is satisfying to one will be exciting to another. Like beauty, it is in the eye of the beholder. Adventure need not always involve climbing mountains or exploring wild terrain. Travelling on a sailing dinghy at sea, or gently canoeing along the local river, may be *your* Mount Everest or North Pole. Excitement should be realised, irrespective of the activity. With adventure comes a desire for learning and finding out. We might say:

Adventure→Excitement→Stimulation→Motivation

Adventure education was developed by *Outward Bound*, whose founder – the late Kurt Haan – stressed the development of an individual's inner resources through physical as well as mental challenges. He began his own adventure school at Aberdovey, designing a thirty-day course in survival for young sailors during World War II. These sailors said they were 'Outward Bound' – headed for challenge and adventure. Since then the movement has expanded considerably, both in Britain and elsewhere throughout the world.

But can adventure be safe? Clearly it must be, although completely to remove the risk element is both impossible and undesirable. But the risks should be controlled as far as possible and no one should develop adventure programmes if they do not feel confident and capable in their activities. People and resources are both important in establishing the quality and safety of the adventure activity, and it is better not to proceed at all than to proceed without caution. Whether we speak of swimming or fishing, rock-climbing or caving, this is still true, and some apparently highly adventurous activities may be made far safer than others, which at first appearance are seemingly tame.

What are the benefits of adventure activities? In their book, *An Introduction to Adventure* (1981), Chris Roland and Mark Havens list twelve.

Activities are essentially non-competitive; there is the challenge of the unknown, creating a high level of involvement and enthusiasm and a sense of accomplishment. Active participation is required by everyone. It promotes co-operation and trust between participants; the entire group communicating and working together to achieve specific goals. Experiences can be implemented at the ability level of participants, enhancing self-concept. Controlled amounts of physical and mental stress can be applied, helping everyone meet challenges presented later in real life situations. Members are respected for trying and involvement, rather than for success or failure. Activities improve relationships between members of the group; one learns to understand the needs and abilities of each other. Outdoor adventure requires co-operation with the elements of nature and a deeper understanding of the environment. Academic skills can be developed in subject areas which are traditionally classroom based. Adventure can lead to better integration of the handicapped participant into society. Everyone can find it enjoyable – and actually have fun.

We clearly see here an opportunity to develop a programme of social education which meets all the requirements of the individual in society. Personal relationships, self-concept, confidence, endeavour, achievement . . . it is all there. How often we hear these words expressed by educationalists, not only about the handicapped individual but concerning the development of young people generally. Adventure education should be for all, but why has the disabled person been neglected or ignored? Perhaps the over-protection afforded by parents, teachers and others responsible for the welfare of handicapped young people has had a great influence in this respect. Perhaps we are all only just becoming aware of what is possible for many disabled individuals. Perhaps the disabled person himself is only now realising what he can do and, more importantly, would like to do! Either way, adventure and the out of door environment are now commonplace in the lives of many who are disabled, and this situation can only improve.

What is possible?

Just about everything – although clearly some outdoor pursuits are easier to organise than others when we are concerned with disability. Some are more suitable for the mentally retarded individual. Yet we find in practice that, with determination and adaptability, most things are possible for most people. Some activities have been available for many years to those who are handicapped. Riding, swimming, camping have all been around for a long time and available as recreational outlets to individuals of many disabilities. Certain activities are of very recent origin and only pursued by a minority – sand and land yachting, ski-bobbing or parascending. In the study organised by the Disabled Living Foundation on sport and physical recreation for mentally handicapped people, Kay Latto found wide evidence of outdoor pursuits being undertaken with trainees from Adult Training Centres, patients from subnormality hospital units, and mentally handicapped school pupils. Sailing and canoeing; rockclimbing and caving; riding and fishing – these are but a few of the activities she refers to in her book *Give Us the Chance* (1981). Whether it is a gentle ramble through summer woods or a winter expedition into the mountains of Wales, there is great adventure for those who usually lead very restricted and protected lives in the highly structured environment of school or hospital.

Where do we begin?

Initially perhaps we should think simply about activities. There is much that can be done out of doors without costly facilities, special resources or highly trained staff. Transport, too, might prove a problem if large numbers were involved. Often these limitations can become the reason for *not* doing things, but what a pity! Rambles close to home, weekend camps, night hikes, a cycle ride, are all very easy to arrange and will take everyone out into open countryside. Even in the city and urban environment things are possible, for there are always extensive parks and open ground, and most can be reached by public transport. In London there are so many rural spaces that one can be even better situated than in more isolated locations. How easy to take the Underground and arrive at Hampstead Heath, or the London Transport bus to Epping Forest! So begin at home . . . look about you and see what is available. In this way you will at least venture outside, and you will find that so much enjoyment is gained by everyone that the idea must be worth expanding. The ramble leads to the hike, the weekend camp to longer adventures, and perhaps a sledge on the local slopes will lead to a full winter sports holiday.

Many special schools, hospitals for mentally handicapped people and residential centres are sited miles from anywhere, remote from town and city and with extensive grounds. In my previous book, *Out of doors with Handicapped People* (1981) I described ways in which these could be used for environmental education and leisure, but they can also be developed for adventure. In America many camps and outdoor centres have built roped adventure courses which were designed with the handicapped person in mind. These are described by Chris Roland and Mark Havens and anyone wanting to consider the use of their grounds in this manner would be well advised to consult their book and follow its practical advice. Simple materials are used – ropes, tyres, planking, poles, and special skills such as balance, confidence and perseverence are developed. The courses are also great fun! Many aspects of outdoor adventure can be learned in your own grounds. Simple map reading and orienteering; use of a compass – where possible; camp craft – cooking, erecting tents, 'backwoods skills' and one-night camps. Survival, safety and first aid can all be introduced in this way and may provide activities for winter months or evenings. Don't feel that outdoor activities should be confined simply to summer days! Many of our linked activities, referred to later, can be practised out of season.

Eventually you will want to move further away, but again utilise your nearby facilities. A local river, lake or canal gives further opportunities for hikes, as well as permitting you to introduce fishing, canoeing or perhaps sailing. If a dinghy is not available, try an inflatable; if that is impossible use a canoe. Wherever possible, link up with a local club, school or college for facilities and expertise. Do not be afraid to approach them. In my own experience most people are willing to help if you only ask. Riding can always be arranged locally and if you find a centre which is approved by Riding for the Disabled, then help will be on hand together with horses and equipment. Saddles, hard hats, mounting blocks . . . and experience. You will find your task much easier. Some of our adventure activities are highly specialised, requiring precise staffing skills and costly equipment, and are only really possible in certain locations. Rock climbing, caving, skiing, mountaineering, perhaps represent the ultimate adventure challenges and will never be available to everyone. Often they will be single experiences, never to be repeated. But how often is this true for all of us, handicapped or able bodied? We must never under-estimate the value of such experiences – the part they play in developing our confidence, showing our qualities of leadership and determination and in helping mould our personality.

Active holidays
An introduction to the more adventurous outdoor pursuits is perhaps best found in an active holiday. Specialised centres now provide for both mentally retarded and physically disabled individuals of all ages, while some outdoor centres, normally catering for a more able population, have now designed facilities to allow use by handicapped participants. Many clubs organise active holidays – The Gateway Club, PHAB, and other similar organisations. Riding holidays are arranged by the Riding for the Disabled Association; the Uphill Ski Club and British Ski Club for the Disabled can be found each year in the winter resorts of Austria, France,

Switzerland or Italy, with active young people of wide-ranging disabilities. Cruising holidays are possible on canals, rivers and at sea, and can be arranged through normal tourist agencies or direct, by reference to advertisements in newspapers and magazines. Canoe camps are held for handicapped children and adolescents each year on the River Tamar. Many charitable organisations based on specific disabilities (the Spastics Society; ASBAH: Mencap; the Muscular Dystrophy Group) arrange holidays or will give advice on holidays. The Tourist Boards are also in contact with establishments providing active holidays which may be suitable for handicapped people; and the Royal Association for Disability and Rehabilitation (RADAR) publishes an annual guide, *The holidays for the physically handicapped guide*, which has a section devoted to active outdoor holidays.

Such holiday weeks can provide the opportunity to tackle rockclimbing or sailing, canoeing or riding, skiing or sub-aqua, with specialist staff and all the resources necessary on hand. While costs may sometimes seem high, it is still easier and less expensive than trying to provide your own facilities. The added advantage is that everybody on the holiday can try several activities, and this will give some indication of just how successful each venture can be. Perhaps the specialist centres are best able to give this range of opportunities at a competitive price. They also have the expertise which comes from many years of arranging courses for handicapped people with wide ranging problems and limitations. In this respect the Churchtown Farm Field Studies Centre in Cornwall, and the Calvert Trust Adventure Centre in Cumbria, are perhaps best able to meet the demands of a specialised population.

In my earlier book I described Churchtown Farm in some detail, and reference is also made by Kay Latto to its courses and their success with mentally handicapped trainees. This centre is able to introduce a wide range of adventure activities to an equally wide range of visitors. No one is too handicapped to attend a course, and each week is designed specifically for the group or individuals attending. The course may include many activities or may be based on a selected theme – sailing, cruising, riding, canoeing. Groups attend from schools and colleges, hospitals and residential homes, training centres and clubs. The participants include those who are blind or deaf; those physically disabled or mentally retarded; the multiply handicapped and emotionally disturbed; the young and the old – in fact everybody! The centre is open throughout the year and the relatively mild (but wet) climate allows courses to operate from January until December. In considering such an active holiday due attention should be given to the lower costs of travel and accommodation out of the high season period.

The Calvert Trust Centre, near Keswick, looks out over the waters of Bassenthwaite, below the mountain range of Skiddaw in the English Lake District. Accommodation is partly in a large, old stone house, and partly in converted outbuildings. Because of winter conditions the courses mainly operate from March until late October, although leisure activities may be available out of season. The variety of adventure pursuits is similar to those offered at Churchtown Farm – sailing, canoeing, riding, fishing, climbing and hiking. Both centres have warm, indoor swimming pools for leisure and canoe instruction. Very recently, the Calvert Trust have established a second centre, with similar functions, in the Kielder Forest, Northumberland.

In Northern Ireland an activity centre for handicapped people became the aim of an organisation called SHARE and was realised during the International Year of Disabled People. Integration is the key in the philosophy of SHARE and, as well as providing integrated active holidays, with canoeing, sailing, fishing and riding, it is intended to give employment, work experience and training to young people both handicapped and able bodied. Located on the shores of Upper Lough Erne, in County Fermanagh, outdoor facilities appear to be excellent.

Existing outdoor centres have in some cases been modified to accommodate small groups of handicapped visitors. One such establishment is the Low Mill Youth Centre, at Askrigg, in the Yorkshire Dales National Park. Close to lake and moor, it is well sited for specialised activities such as caving, and use is made of the North Craven and Swaledale systems.

Linked activities

A feature of courses at Churchtown Farm is the linking together of physical adventure activities with teaching in environmental subjects. Much of its success can be attributed to this aspect of life, since the learning processes are stimulated by the atmosphere created in adventure. It can be highly exciting to hike over a wild moor in winter, but in addition this provides a perfect setting for finding out about rocks and landscape, climate and vegetation. Bogs and their mosses are so much more meaningful in wet weather, and the habits of winter-visiting birds are better understood when you see them yourself, rather than only hearing of them from books or television. In summer, it is a marvellous experience to canoe close to the edge of a rocky shore on a low spring tide and watch anemones waving tentacles and crabs crawling among seaweed-covered crevices. At sea we can learn about waves and tides, tow a net to sample the surface-living plankton or watch gannets and terns plummeting deep in penetrating dives. Irrespective of the environment or time of year there is always something to observe, and minds are so much more stimulated under these conditions. Often staff, attending with their handicapped trainees or pupils, would say how successful the educational aspects of a course had been even if they had travelled originally to follow a more active based programme; and that their mentally retarded youngsters had seemed to learn more in a week than they had over many previous years. Of course, this is essentially only the result of intensive stimulation. The right environment; the right atmosphere; the right results! What a pity that we cannot create this situation for more children – and adults – in more places and over longer periods. Learning should be fun and an enjoyable experience for both staff and pupils.

Every adventure activity described in the following chapters of this book can form the basis and create the ideal environment for learning. Many suitable topics and methods of presentation can be found in my earlier book, to which frequent references will be made, for I sincerely believe that they must be used together. The one creates the adventure mood; the other shows how to utilise it.

1   In the water

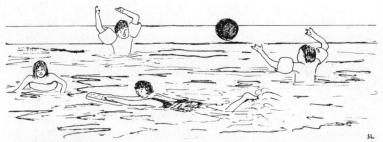

Introduction

Swimming is often considered to be an essential first stage in participation in various water sports, especially canoeing and sailing. So while not necessarily an outdoor adventure activity itself, we should consider its role in leading on to other things. Swimming is usually introduced to youngsters in the confines of a heated pool, but we must always remember that the open river or sea is a very different and more hostile environment. Indeed, while some swimmers can cope in the pool they will fail in open waters, due not only to the lower temperature there but also to the vast expanse of water presented especially at sea. Currents and tides also play a highly important part in self-survival in large rivers and at sea, while wild, swirling waters will often deter the capsized canoeist.

However, swimming is probably the most popular leisure activity introduced to children at a young age, whether they are handicapped or not, and water as a therapeutic medium is an essential part of the lifestyle of physically disabled young people. In the hydrotherapy situation the pool temperature often approaches body temperature – 98.4°F (37°C) – and physiotherapists find that for complete relaxation those with severe neuro-motor handicaps, such as muscular dystrophy and spasticity, require water at this temperature or above. However, the hydrotherapy pool is usually too warm and comfortable to teach swimming and a lower temperature of about 86°F (30°C) is desirable for physically disabled youngsters. Seldom are public pools kept at this temperature and they will often be found to be too cold – 80°F (27°C) – for many who are disabled, although suitable for many mentally retarded swimmers. Of course the swimmer generates his own body heat, which the learner standing in shallow water fails to do, and pool sessions are best kept to short periods of about fifteen minutes for such beginners. Similarly, the more severely physically handicapped persons will rapidly cool in pool waters and may be unable to communicate this to their helpers who consequently must remember regularly to ask this question of their partners. The pool must remain enjoyable to the beginner and even though many will never learn to swim unaccompanied, the fun situation and water experience should not be denied them. Indeed, water represents the ideal medium for the severely handicapped person, allowing him or her to leave behind the wheelchair and leg-irons, forget the contortions of an often deformed body and float, relaxed in a buoyant environment.

Swimming sessions

Although many schools catering for handicapped pupils have their own swimming pool, there are many others that have to go to the local leisure centre or other public pool. Adult training centres, residential centres and handicapped individuals must all rely for their swim on public pools, unless a local college or similar institution has a pool which can be acquired for a session. Often clubs, such as the Gateway, PHAB, and other local leisure and recreation clubs for disabled participants, will organise pool sessions in their area, which will be cheaper and have staff and volunteers arranged for your assistance. If you wish to arrange such a session then the leisure centre or pool manager will usually be only too happy to assist and to suggest suitably qualified instructors.

High staff ratios are necessary and most would agree that each handicapped swimmer or beginner should ideally have his or her own helper, who will not be a qualified instructor but who relates well to the handicapped partner and helps to develop confidence in the water. The helper also confirms the safety of his or her handicapped partner. The instructor should be free to move between pairs to teach techniques and check on safety.

It is also essential that at least one competent swimmer, preferably with a life-saving qualification (Royal Life Saving Society Bronze Medallion) or at least with training in rescue methods and in resuscitation, remains at the side of the pool all the time and keeps a constant surveillance over all participants. The life-guard should not enter the water, except to effect a rescue, and he should always carry a whistle to draw attention to any person in difficulties. He should be aware of all handicapped people in the water who have special problems, such as epilepsy, and should be able to deal with anyone having a convulsion. Quite frequently a group of mentally retarded or cerebral palsied swimmers will include members who are also epileptic and a special watch should be maintained over their safety in the water. The size of the group at any time should not exceed the safety limits set by the instructor and one should remember that most pairs will remain in shallow waters, thus reducing the total effective area of pool available to the group.

Sufficient helpers must be available to help in changing and drying handicapped swimmers, since many will need two helpers, especially if the swimmer is normally confined to a wheelchair. It is true to say that however many helpers you have, you never have enough!

Helpers too need instruction, especially in the handling of their charges and in coping with particular problems (such as communication limitations, deafness, behavioural problems, epilepsy), as well as in techniques to develop water confidence and to allow maximum participation by their handicapped partner. The Amateur Swimming Association (ASA) is the official body giving certificate awards to those successfully completing their training courses. Instructors should hold a Swimming Teachers Certificate. The ASA also have a development officer for the disabled and pilot conditions for a Teacher of Disabled Swimmers Certificate and for an Instructor-Aide Certificate for Disabled Swimmers. Both the ASA and the Swimming Teachers Association (STA) produce schemes with badges and certificates awarded for swimmers completing each stage. These may be distance awards or based on personal survival.

Water confidence

In the early days of introducing mentally handicapped and physically disabled people to the pool environment it is important to approach the activity slowly, in a series of gradual stages. Clearly it may be easier to introduce swimming to children, rather than adults, but then this may be equally true for everyone. It may be sufficient to establish water confidence for the handicapped person, prior to introducing him or her to other water sports, such as canoeing and sailing, but this should be tested in cold water situations before the individual is allowed out onto open water. A lifejacket, or buoyancy aid, can also be tested on a particular individual, both to see how effective it is for some types of disability and in addition to find out how the individual will react when alone in the water, supported only by the aid and not by the comforting hands of a helper.

Indeed, the whole subject of flotation aids is of interest, since they can certainly be used to develop water confidence; although many feel that once the candidate feels dependent on his support systems it becomes exceedingly difficult, if not impossible, gradually to remove them. However, in group situations, especially where each swimmer is not accompanied by his or her own helper, flotation aids are important to safety, and most learning and fun sessions will certainly include handicapped youngsters wearing either arm bands or waist rings or both. Arm bands should be of an approved design, with safety valves and preferably double-chambered, since if one side loses air the other continues to give support. Full inflation can gradually lead to reduced inflation once confidence is established, and especially if the individual is beginning to swim. Arm bands should fit securely over the upper arm but not be too tight. They can be worn alone. Rubber waist rings keep the abdomen near to the water surface but should not be worn alone since the individual can slip from inside the ring. In this event the ring tends to come over the arms and head, slipping from beneath the armpits. The wearing of arm bands will help prevent this and provide a supplementary safety system.

The method of entry into the water will vary according to the degree of disability. While most mentally retarded swimmers can enter the pool via the steps, care being taken over pool balance in many instances, the more severely physically disabled swimmers will require lifting from the wheelchair into the water. Some special pools, designed for use by disabled people, may have a ramp direct into the water down which a shower chair can be wheeled and the person floated out into the pool. Another design is the raised pool, where the walls are at the same height as the seat of a wheelchair and the disabled swimmer can transfer laterally from the chair to the top of the tiled wall of the pool. They can then be lowered by helpers already in the water. In all instances, staff must be both on the pool side and in the water to transfer candidates from one side to the other.

Once in the water, confidence will be gradually gained by the helper talking to his partner, moving about in the water, maintaining constant proximity to the sides and not making sudden movements or demands on his charge. It may be enough merely to sit on the steps, dabbling feet in the water, and gradually moving down the steps until one is sitting with water around the waist or chest. Each participant will behave as an individual, and what is true for one will be false for another. After a time one can introduce the handicapped person to 'getting the face wet' and 'water in the eyes'. Both can be fearful experiences and most young people do not like this, whether handicapped or very able! Play is important here – washing faces with wet hands, blowing bubbles in the water surface, very gentle splashing, creating waves. Often the participant will cling to the helper, and body contact is important. If the helper finds his partner is very tense, clinging tightly and generally unhappy it is certain that one has progressed 'too far too soon'. Water confidence can take a very long time to develop!

Water fun
Visiting the pool should be looked upon as fun – pure and simple enjoyment. Any benefits, therapeutic or sporting, are secondary and this should not be forgotten by organisers and helpers. The novelty of going will soon wear off unless the participant enjoys it all, and in any case the stimulated youngster or trainee is far more likely to be taught to swim.

There are many water games that can be introduced, some more suitable for children but others designed for the older group. Once again it will depend on the degree of disability in the group – mentally retarded trainees can participate in ball games, use polystyrene floats and move about quite actively. The more physically disabled individual will often need to rely on the physical support of the helper and the games will then be very different.

An excellent programme of such games is given in a publication by the Association of Swimming Therapy, *Swimming for the Disabled* (1981). The games are graded in difficulty and fourteen are illustrated and described, indicating the position and role of the helper in each case. Each game has a name – bicycles, rag dolls, snake, spaceships – and anyone planning a programme for handicapped swimmers should read this book.

The advantage of group games, in addition to pure fun, is that the 'helper-swimmer' partnership can gradually be reduced in intensity, since the swimmer begins to relate to the group as a whole for support rather than to a single person. Eventual release of hands from the body of the swimmer may well come about through such games. Similarly, within the group aids can be dispensed with provided there are as many helpers as handicapped swimmers. Music and song can also be used within many games – why not take a battery tape recorder along to your next pool session?

Swimming methods

There will be many misconceptions about what is meant by the term 'swimming' with respect to handicapped people. Some who are mentally retarded and the less physically disabled may acquire traditional stroke skills and swim by front or back crawl or by breaststroke. For them the pool is an opening to a beneficial leisure activity; or to competitive swimming in such functions as the Special Olympics, or in local, national and international galas arranged for specific groups of handicapped swimmers or for disabled participants in general. But for many others swimming will remain an act of self-propulsion through the water, using untraditional stroke methods, often with one region of the body not participating in movement, and with the permanent aid of flotation devices. Some will never attain self-propulsion without the helper on hand to give friendly support, either psychological or physical, but will still gain enormous benefit from their swimming sessions.

Many swimming teachers, in schools and clubs, now utilise the effective Halliwick method, first introduced by James McMillan in 1949, at the school of the same name. It is based on the physical properties of water and on the ways in which an object will behave when placed in water. Thus it takes into account density, the centre of gravity, flotation, buoyancy, forces and turbulence. These, together with a detailed description of the method, are best learned by reading the book *'Swimming for the Disabled'* which is based entirely on Halliwick. Courses are organised on a regional basis – usually over a weekend – and details of them can be obtained from the Association of Swimming Therapy (AST). There is also a film, called *Water Free*, presented by the AST, which in 35 minutes describes the Halliwick method.

Swimmers are taught on a one-to-one ratio, without the use of aids, until the time when complete independence is achieved. Correct handling by the helper is important and several holds are described, giving 'face to face' contact as well as the often used 'back float' position. With progression the helper gradually reduces support, from firm holds to lighter waist support and to the horizontal position where the swimmer floats on his back, with his neck supported by the shoulder of the upright helper. The helper then walks backwards, with his partner either floating in a still position or kicking with the legs. Swimmers are made familiar with conceivable body rotations and how to react to control such movements. Also how to breathe safely in the water with the face clear of the surface, how to regain such a position and how to control breathing-out when water covers the face.

Other methods of instruction can be designed by individual swimming instructors, and one such system is described by Kay Latto, in her book *Give Us The Chance* (1981). Designed by an ASA club-coach who was also concerned with the team for the Special Olympics in New York, it is particularly appropriate for mentally handicapped children and trainees. Play is a way of learning, and it encourages activities involving physical and mental effort. It also relies on aids to enable swimmers to experience the sensation of moving in water in a horizontal position as soon as possible. Each person has both a ring and arm bands, and during later stages extra aids such as foot flippers and floats are used. It also states that swimmers often ask to swim without aids when they are ready, after which they are told that air is being let out from arm bands and the ring. On first swimming without aids they should move towards the pool edge, across an imaginary 'river', and progress by widening the river. Throughout the early stages the swimmer is buoyed in the water and any aids that can assist in flotation, leg kicking and other movements are encouraged.

Clearly the two methods are very different in principle and technique, but both are appropriate for introducing handicapped people to the world of water, and providing the method is safe and enjoyable the end result will be very similar.

Snorkels and sub-aqua

Although clearly not activities for everybody, there are many disabled swimmers who are capable of finding adventure underwater. Equipped with a face mask and breathing tube, and wearing flippers on the feet if possible, the snorkel diver is able to move with ease below the water surface, either at sea or in lakes and rivers. Practice should of course be gained earlier in the pool, and many swimming clubs will advise both on courses which are available and where to buy your gear.

If you enjoy the fun that can be had from these sports, then you will soon need a wet suit, and it is often possible to obtain one second-hand from someone who has perhaps outgrown his own. The wet suit can be used for your other adventure sports, such as canoeing and sailing, so it may well be money worth spending. Incidentally, even very cold waters do not seem so bad when you are dressed in a good wet suit of appropriate gauge. There are several styles, and tops can be bought with or without arms and worn in conjunction with separate trousers and rubber socks. Alternatively flippers can be worn on the bare feet. For the disabled person the added protection against skin abrasion and low temperatures can be given by a wet suit. Extra thickness can be given to knees and elbows by 'pads' cemented onto the normal suit, and suitable off-cuts of material can usually be purchased from manufacturers of wet suits.

When you buy the face mask and snorkel beware of cheap productions. The face plate should be shatterproof and the mask must seal properly and cover eyes and nose. The snorkel must not be more than eighteen inches (46cm) long, separate from the mask, j-shaped and with a good smooth mouth-piece (BS 4532 1969).

Armed with a rubber-armoured, weatherproof camera (Minolta) which is waterproof in the upper few metres, you will be able to enjoy your 'dives' and bring photographs home for the collection. What a way to spend a future holiday!

Few will extend their interest to full sub-aqua diving, but although a minority sport, it is a real adventure for some who are physically disabled. Norman Croucher, in his book *Outdoor Pursuits for Disabled People* (1981), refers to some paraplegics, who normally use wheelchairs, being trained over a five day period and participating in marine dives. Amputees, deaf and blind people can also be considered as potential divers. Certain categories of handicap – epilepsy, diabetes, those involving the respiratory system and heart, certain types of deafness, hypertension – will prohibit sub-aqua diving, but it is the policy of the British Sub-Aqua Club to encourage branches to accept disabled members. A medical report should be obtained by anyone anticipating this activity, and the club will give guidelines to the medical practitioner. If the disabled diver is unable to undertake rescues then he should always dive with at least two others who are able-bodied. The coaching scheme will determine whether, and at what stage, a disabled diver can move from the pool to open water situations.

The British Sub-Aqua Club produces manuals for both diving and snorkelling, and the revised edition of *Water Sports for the Disabled* (1983) will give the most up-to-date information on both activities.

2 Life afloat

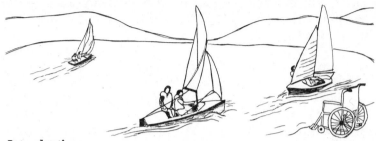

Introduction

Terry was enjoying himself. He could see the squall approaching as the dark grey cloud scuttled towards him. Heavy rain sheeted down to the sea and sharp gusts of wind ruffled the water surface in a wide arc.

'Batten the hatches!' he piped in his squeaky voice. No one stirred.

'Splice the mainbrace!' Still no reaction.

'There's a thing coming, look!' Terry jerked his arm towards the squall. Heads and bodies rotated to look. Mutters and exclamations were heard from the crew ranged along the sides of the longboat.

'Hoods up! Stand by the sheets!' A brief flurry of activity ensued as anorak hoods were pulled up and holds tightened on the jib sheets, main sheet and mizzen sheet.

'Is it in or out?' enquired Robert, a little anxiously.

'Er . . .' Terry darted a glance at the skipper by his side. The skipper returned the enquiring glance, not very helpfully. We're on starboard tack, thought Terry, shifting his calipered legs to a more comfortable position, so with the wind blowing out from the centre, it'll blow more into the sails. That'll try to push us over, so if we loosen the sails, we'll keep upright.

'Is that right?' he asked.

'Sorry,' replied the skipper, 'were you muttering to yourself?'

'Oh, loosen – I mean out,' said Terry hopefully. 'A bit,' he added, to cover himself.

The squall drew closer, soft gusts of wind and splutters of rain reaching ahead of the ruffled arc of water. Just as the disturbed wavelets reached the longboat, Terry shouted, 'Now!' and ducked his head as the driving rain splattered heavily into his face. The boat tipped suddenly to port, then slowly straightened up as the sails were let out and the rolling motion stayed. The forward jib sail whipped out and flapped wildly in the strong wind.

'James, you let go again!' Terry screeched.

'It slipped!' the plaintive wail floated back on the wind.

Margaret, sitting forward to port, helped retrieve the jib sheet with her good hand and passed it across the boat to James.

'Don't let me fall,' James counselled, as he slid down the seat. By his side Mr Jenkins kept a firm grip on his shoulders as James reached across to grasp the proffered rope with his toes and struggled back to a sitting position. He then deftly pulled the sheet taut and hauled the jib tighter until the flapping ceased.

'That's fine!' called Terry, grinning with delight as the rain coursed down his face and dribbled off his nose.

'Blow the man down, bullies, blow the man down,' Miss Davis burst into song with gusto.

'Off! Off!'

'Oh, Miss!'

'Throw her overboard!' and other cries of derision drowned the shouts of 'More!' and 'Well done, Miss Davis,' from the skipper and Mr Jenkins.

The squall passed over as quickly as it had arrived. The wind backed and lessened, and bright sunshine replaced the rain. The sails started to flap.

'Haul in the sheets!' called Terry. 'Cor, that was great. Would anyone else like to take the helm?'

Cries of 'Me!' 'It's my turn!' and 'I want a go!' burst forth as Terry relinquished the tiller to the skipper. He shuffled along the seat to make way for the next eager helmsman, feeling very pleased with himself.

Sailing opportunities

Sailing is an activity enjoyed by an increasingly large number of people from all walks of life. Once a pastime reserved for a minority of privileged enthusiasts, the past twenty years have been a boom time for the sport. Many inland sailing areas have been made available by local Water Authorities and the Water

Space Amenity Commission, from whom information may be obtained. The number of marinas has grown, and the number of sailing clubs has mushroomed.

During the last ten years the Royal Yachting Association has been instrumental in promoting opportunities for introducing sailing to beginners, improving individuals' performance, and co-ordinating the work of sailing and yachting clubs.

The RYA is actively encouraging clubs to integrate disabled people on an individual basis. Energetic complementary roles are being played by the National School Sailing Association and the Water Sports Division, British Sports Association for the Disabled. Together these organisations are providing effective comprehensive opportunities for sailing for people who are physically disabled. On a much smaller scale, in terms of organisation if not monetary expenditure, other bodies are making vital contributions.

The 45-foot catamaran *Sparkle* was purpose-built for wheel-chair users by SPARKS, Sportsmen Pledged to Aid Research into Crippling. Several specially refitted narrow boats are available for hire by groups of handicapped people. The RYA Seamanship Foundation holds cruising courses for blind people and can supply details about the trimaran *Challenger*, a stable craft used by disabled people. The Jubilee Sailing Trust has been formed to design, build and operate a 127-foot sail training ship, *The Lord Nelson*, to accommodate a trainee crew of 45 physically disabled and able-bodied people.

Aids and adaptations to craft and equipment are continually being innovated, mostly at a local level as the need arises. However, a device with more universal application is the 'Sailsafe Sailing Seat'. This was designed by Emlyn Davies to enable severely disabled people to steer and race sailing dinghies. The seat is well proven and widely used, but, like most devices, it is not perfect. The seat is heavy, cumbersome and, when not in use, is in the way. The sailsafe seat is obtainable from *Newton Aids Ltd, Unit 4, Dolphin Industrial Estate, Southampton Road, Salisbury, Wiltshire.*

Physically disabled people now have nearly as much access to sailing as do able-bodied people. The limitations imposed are not excessive. A disabled boat owner may need to acquire two crew instead of one. He may need assistance in launching and recovering his boat, but then so do most sailors. Even single-handed sailing is enjoyed by a number of disabled enthusiasts. There is, however, room for improvement in the number of land-based sailing facilities providing access for wheel-chairs.

Opportunities for mentally handicapped and multiply handicapped people to participate in sailing are considerably more limited, and rarely initiated by sailing organisations. But there are several organisations and establishments for mentally handicapped children and adults who make their own arrangements at a local level. These are usually initiated by members of staff who are themselves sailing enthusiasts. However, sailing can be organised by staff and parents who know nothing about sailing but do have an intimate knowledge of their son or daughter, or the students or patients in their care.

Sailing or boating can be a marvellous experience for anyone, at any level. For people who are mentally retarded, the level of excitement, enjoyment and the fine line between adventure and misadventure, can be judged most exactly by a parent, member of staff or instructor who knows each individual well. The activity can and should be pitched at a level most suited to the needs, temperament, abilities and disabilities of each individual to achieve the optimum success and satisfaction.

Therefore, unless the instructor is very experienced in boating with handicapped people, he will not do himself justice, nor satisfy the needs of his students, without considerable assistance from the parents or staff. An intimate knowledge of the emotional, physical and medical idiosyncrasies of the individual student is most desirable – even if this knowledge is acquired at second-hand.

Sailing for mentally handicapped students should not be restricted to instructing the 'RYA Method'. Although a suitable formula for teaching non-handicapped beginners to sail, for many handicapped students this may not be at all desirable. Rather, the aim should be to emulate Water Rat in his sheer joy of 'simply messing about in boats'. This should be borne in mind when considering suitable instructors, craft, equipment and safety measures.

What to wear

Yachting boots; or neoprene boots; or plimsolls and thick
   socks.

Socks: thick, woollen.

Trousers: warm, wool or cotton, and loose.

Shirt: warm, wool or cotton.

Sweaters: thick, woollen or thermal.

Underwear: cotton, wool or thermal vests if prone to the cold.

Waterproofs: one-piece suit or anorak and overtrousers; wind
   and water proof.

Gloves: wool, thermal or waterproof.

Headgear: wool hat or balaclava.

Staff

Ideally the staff would comprise the skipper or sailing
instructor, an experienced crew, and other staff (houseparents,
teachers and parents for example) to increase the staff: student
ratio to 1:1. The ratio may be increased or decreased depending
on the abilities of the individual students, type of craft, weather
conditions and the sailing area. In principle, the higher the
potential risk, the higher the staff:student ratio. It should be
appreciated that the lower the ratio, the less effective the
teaching will probably be.

The staff responsible for the students must be completely
open and honest with the instructor about any problems they
may have. Staff can be very coy about revealing the extent of
their charges' handicaps lest any be excluded from participating
in the sailing activity. Any secrecy could put an individual or
the whole group at risk. In one incident a mentally retarded
young man, seeking attention, threw a self-induced fit, and in
doing so unintentionally knocked himself out on a hatch cover.
The only member of staff who knew of his propensity was in
another boat. The young man recovered with no ill effects, but
any danger could have been avoided by appointing a forewarned
staff member to stay by him prepared and ready to assist him if
necessary.

People prone to bouts of hysteria, if manifested in a violent
way, need to be closely controlled, and it would be preferable
for them, as well as poorly-controlled epileptics, to sail in a
large craft rather than a small dinghy. Hydrophobia sufferers

should not be taken in a boat which has any measurable chance of capsizing: the consequential panic could have dire consequences, but in any case it is unlikely that such a person would willingly choose to sail in such a craft; better for all if a cruise in a substantial vessel was chosen instead.

All members of staff need to be constantly vigilant, not only in terms of seamanship but also to assess and respond to the needs and behaviour of the students.

The suitable instructor would have a broad and extensive knowledge of sailing and boating, with a wealth of experience behind him. It would be desirable to hold the RYA Dayboat Instructor Award or the RYA/DOT Coastal Skipper Certificate. He needs to be adaptable and flexible in his approach both to boating and instructing, and, when with handicapped people, should sail well within his own capabilities. This may include, for example, reefing much earlier than he would normally. It would be very helpful to have a sound knowledge of the sailing area to be used. The instructor will be more effective as an instructor if he is given the opportunity to gain the confidence of the students, and to get to know them as individuals.

The skipper carries a heavy burden of responsibility which is considerably eased by the presence of a reliable and knowledgeable crew. Contact with instructors can be made through the RYA, the National School Sailing Association, sailing and yachting clubs and county outdoor pursuits organisers.

The enjoyment of the students can be greatly enhanced by those staff who are not sailors. We all have some skills and knowledge to offer and those of the non-sailors can complement to advantage the sailing skills of the skipper and crew. A small boat is unique in being, if only for a short time, a vessel or island holding a small self-contained community within which all experiences are shared. The staff can turn this situation to advantage to encourage the handicapped students to become involved and play a real role in this community. The learning of physical skills and social skills can be taught effectively within the community. The whole unit can also be moved en masse from one field studies location to another. Teachers have a captive audience within a movable classroom.

What type of boat?
The choice of craft may depend on your location; whether the sailing is to be a 'one-off' experience, a frequent, regular activity, or a holiday; and the availability of transport and funds.

There is a multitude of sailing craft to choose from, and any examples given will be to illustrate the type rather than to recommend any particular make. Boats built of glass reinforced plastic (GRP) require much less maintenance than those of traditional timber construction, but additional equipment is not so easy to attach. Plywood boats are generally not as strong as either GRP or timber, although in their favour they are cheaper and can be made up from kit form even less expensively. Thus boat-building could be used as an integral part of the overall boating experience.

The Wayfarer is a 16 foot GRP bermudan rigged sailing dinghy, very popular with sailing schools. It is relatively stable, has good handling characteristics and is very forgiving. There

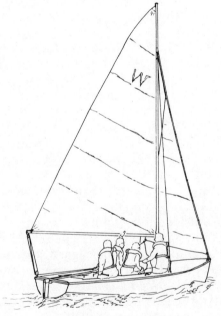

Wayfarer dinghy

is ample capacity for four persons. As with all dinghies the Wayfarer can be capsized, but despite its bulk, is easily righted single handed. For handicapped novices, it may be unwise to use a sailing dinghy less than 14 feet in length unless the students are agile and quick to respond, or the wind and sea conditions are calm.

For beginners with some experience and ability, however, a small dinghy is very good for improving skills. Close supervision is of course essential.

The Optimist is a 7½ foot marine ply or GRP single-sail dinghy specially designed for children up to 16 years and available in kit form.

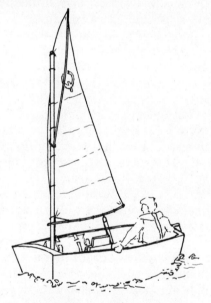

Optimist dinghy

The Mirror Dinghy is an 11 foot gunter rigged dinghy of marine ply available in kit form, suitable for older children, but will carry an adult.

The Tinker Traveller is a sailing inflatable dinghy of strong and safe construction. To correct the wayward tendencies of inflatables caused by their shallow draught, the dagger board is very deep – four feet. This can make things a little tricky if sailing in shallow water. The advantage for disabled sailors is the soft material of inflatables, as mentioned below.

The Topper is a single-sail light-weight plastic dinghy. Designed for single-handed sailing, it is wet and relatively unstable with little head room below the boom. On the plus side, a capsize is not hazardous, and the Topper can be righted in seconds and sailed away without bailing. It is very much a fun boat.

The Optimist, Mirror and Topper are all well established as sound training and international racing dinghies, extensively used by clubs, schools, associations, county councils, regional authorities and individual owners.

Windsurfers, or sailboards, are like surfboards with a single mast and sail attached. They require a unique handling technique needing agility, balance and good limb control. Until skill is acquired, the windsurfer spends as much time in the water as on the board.

The Drascombe Longboat is a 22 foot GRP yawl with provision for an outboard motor. This is a remarkably versatile craft. The open version has ample seating capacity for eight (including skipper and crew), and the cabin model can be provided with toilet, stove and bunks while retaining a very roomy cockpit. The three sails, comprising jib, main and mizzen, can all be reefed. Roller-reefing is available for the jib. The longboat sails well without the mainsail, although performance suffers towards the wind. It does not point very close to the wind anyway, and under mizzen and jib alone a close reach is generally the best that can be achieved. There is no boom to thwack unwary heads, but a standing helmsman can position himself nicely to head the clew tackle as it whizzes past when going about or gybing. The retractable centre-plate can be utilised like that of a dinghy, and together with the removable rudder, facilitates beaching and loading or unloading in shallow water. There are thwarts for rowing. When under power the boat can be steered with the tiller and separately controlled by the instructor using the outboard engine tiller. Thus the student can steer the boat in his own fashion in apparent control, while the instructor, sitting behind the helmsman, can maintain or retrieve complete control by overriding the rudder by means of the outboard motor controls.

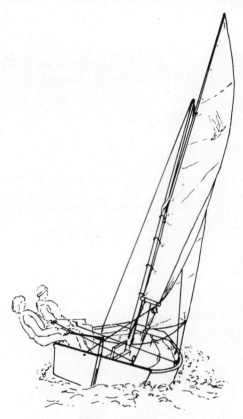

Mirror dinghy

The Drascombe Longboat has room to move about in and is difficult to capsize. It handles well, both under sail or power, and is suitable for inshore waters as well as estuaries and inland waters. For its size, the Longboat is quite easy to trail.

Yachts and motor sailers (designed to sail under engine and sail together), have advantages similar to the Drascombe Longboat, and in addition are more comfortable for extended cruises. Characteristics which may be disadvantages are: high freeboard may make boarding awkward; cockpits take up only a small proportion of the overall length, and will therefore either be cramped, or accommodate a smaller number of people; the draught is deeper, which limits the places available for landing, or necessitates a tender, which in turn may preclude some disabled people from using the yacht; frequent trailing is impractical if the yacht is large enough for its purpose – if it can be trailed easily, then it is probably too small; the number of suitable locations is severely restricted.

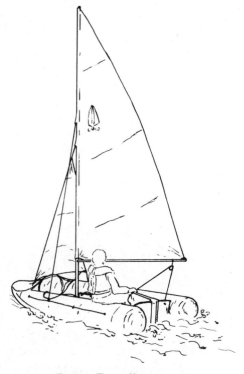

Tinker Traveller

Boating activities with groups of handicapped children or adults need not be confined to sailing boats. A lot of fun, excitement and education can be had from motorised or rowing boats.

Inflatables and semi-inflatables, strongly built, are used by inshore rescue services and by the National Sailing Centre and many sailing clubs for rescue craft. They are very stable and fun to use as a means of transport, for exploration and as a teaching platform. Their shallow draught enables them to go where deep-keeled yachts may not. The soft material of these boats reduces the risk of knocks, cuts and bruises when entering or leaving, and can be more comfortable for some people. Disadvantages: depreciation is high – the life expectancy is only eight years; although rowing is possible, it is very arduous. Properly constructed inflatables complying with British Standard BS MA 16 1971 are very safe, but beware of cheap plastic boats; these are the bane of every rescue service, and many would like to see them banned.

The Dory is a flat open boat having characteristics similar to inflatables, except that it is made of GRP and therefore inflexible but more durable. The Dory is less seaworthy in heavy seas. Dorys are more roomy, size for size, and like inflatables are available in several different lengths.

Motor cruisers, like yachts, come in a variety of shapes, sizes and accommodation. Their main advantage over open boats is the wet weather protection they provide. Few of the smaller cabin cruisers can face the open sea, except in flat calm, and should be used only in sheltered waters.

If you or your organisation intends to purchase a boat, armed with the information contained in this chapter, seek further advice from a knowledgeable sailing friend, or your local yacht or sailing club (which it would be helpful to join), and have potential purchases professionally surveyed. New small craft should be up to the standards of the Ship and Boat Builders' National Federation and larger ones may be certified by Lloyd's surveyors. Remember to reserve enough money to pay for all the essential safety equipment which must be purchased separately.

Safety Equipment
All craft should have a list of things to do and to check before setting sail.

Lifejacket: each person should wear a lifejacket to BS 3595 69 with inherent buoyancy. Each lifejacket should have a whistle securely attached. Within the British Standard specification are a variety of designs, and for individuals it is wise to shop around and try on several types to find one most suitable and comfortable. Children's sizes are also available. Care should be

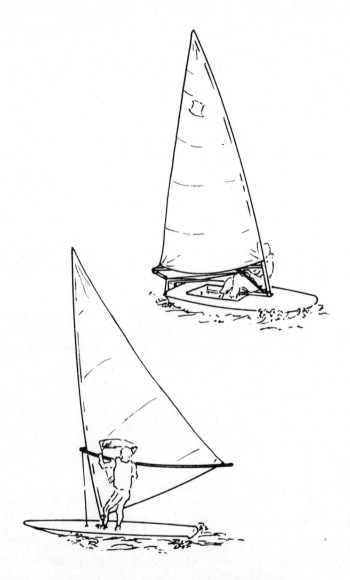

The Topper (*above*); Sailboard (*below*)

taken to ensure the weight limits are adhered to, taking into account heavy aids such as calipers. It should also be borne in mind that even with lifejackets containing inherent buoyancy, the maximum buoyancy of 35 lbs (16 kg) is only achieved when the lifejacket is fully inflated. Similarly lifejackets are designed to turn an inert body onto its back with head held out of the water, only when fully inflated. For most circumstances however, it is practical to keep the lifejacket half-inflated until needed. Further air can be blown in quickly and easily, by a rescuer if necessary. Exceptions are epileptics who would be advised to wear a fully inflated lifejacket at all times when boating. Perhaps the most versatile lifejacket in terms of straps and fastening possibilities is the Ottersport. (For instance the lifting becket can be used as a crutch strap to prevent the lifejacket riding over the head). For an individual's exclusive use, additional straps or alternative fastenings can be added to any otherwise suitable lifejacket. Not all handicapped people can wear lifejackets fitted according to the manufacturer's recommendations. But all lifejackets should be fastened securely and should achieve the position relative to the body as advised by the manufacturer.

Skippers, crews and other staff may prefer to wear a lifejacket without inherent buoyancy. Until inflated, they provide no aid to flotation whatsoever. This means that the wearer can swim underwater if he needs to. This type of lifejacket can be worn flat folded which avoids the problem of restrictive bulk inherent in other lifejackets.

Buoyancy aids: buoyancy aids are aids to flotation and nothing more. They should only be used by people who are very confident in water, and are not recommended for mentally retarded people, or for persons with epilepsy.

Harness: harnesses to BS 4224 or 4474 for children, designed for sailors to secure themselves to the yacht, are essential in extreme weather conditions (which most groups of novice handicapped sailors would never encounter). They could be used, however, to secure hyperactive students or others with a tendency to fall or jump overboard. In small sailing dinghies everyone should be free to fall clear of the boat in the event of a capsize, and should not be attached. Trapezes have a quick-

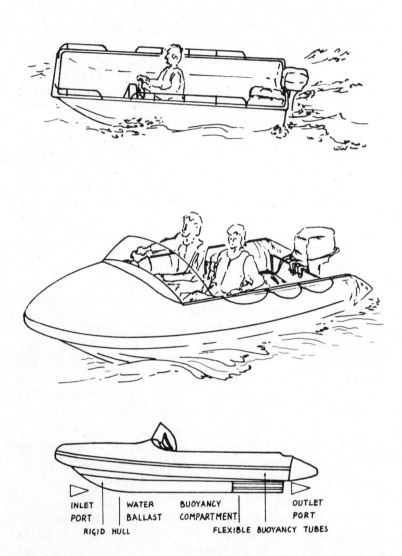

INLET PORT   WATER BALLAST   BUOYANCY COMPARTMENT   OUTLET PORT

RIGID HULL   FLEXIBLE BUOYANCY TUBES

Boating craft: Dory (*above*); Semi-inflatable (*centre and below*)

release attachment, and ought only to be used if the wearer can operate the device quickly and on his own initiative.

Boat Buoyancy: the boat should have enough buoyancy to float upright with its full complement of passengers and crew, when full of water. If this cannot be achieved, then except in extremely safe locations, there should be a liferaft or inflatable tender, or an escort craft or rescue craft in attendance. Each of these, or a combination, should be capable of holding the full complement.

Lifebuoy: for all but the smallest dinghies. The horse-shoe shape is easier to get into than the ring type. Kapok deck cushions can be very useful in an emergency as lifebuoys.

Throw line: this could be a knotted warp, a quoit on a line, or a specially designed throw line. Do test them for suitability before making your choice, and do practise throwing. (This is an activity in which the students could participate.) The line should be buoyant, 100 feet (33m) long and with a minimum breaking strain of 250 lbs (112 kg).

Anchor: this should be of appropriate type and size and length of chain or warp for the type and size of craft and the areas of operation. Where warp is used at least three fathoms of chain should be attached between anchor and warp. Sea going vessels require two anchors.

Bilge pump: for powered craft, the bilge pump should be fixed. On other craft a portable bilge pump which can draw water from the sea may be useful for fire fighting. A bailer or bucket (preferably two) with lanyard should also be carried, or for small dinghies may replace the bilge pump. Self-bailers are not reliable in all weather conditions, and should be considered to be extras.

Distress flares: a minimum of six comprising two red hand flares, two 'two-star' red signals and two orange smoke signals. These are essential at sea and in sheltered waters, and even for some inland waters. More flares with the addition of red parachute rockets are recommended when more than three miles offshore. Most flares have a life expectancy of three years. However, experience has shown that commercially available brand-new flares are as unreliable as time-expired flares. Regrettably a failure rate of one flare out of three has to be expected. To be confident of having enough flares in an emergency, it is prudent to carry twice as many as you envisage needing. This adds up to a lot of expensive flares, which are only to be used if life is endangered. Even if the flares work, they still have to be seen and acted upon to be effective. Since the recent Coastguard reorganisation, there are fewer lookout stations operating and consequently large gaps in visual cover. The Coastguard is relying much more on VHF radio coverage, which forces the yachting fraternity to do the same.

Radio: two-way radios are highly desirable for extended off-shore cruises and are also worth considering if frequent flotilla-type excursions are made. VHF radio should be reserved for contact with the outside world, for coastguard information or distress calls. The user is required to hold a government issued licence. Citizen's Band radios (CB) can be used on inland waters and for less serious messages at sea. Their use would enhance safety within the flotilla, and introduce another valuable educational tool. If radios are not available, a megaphone or loud hailer facilitates communication. For extended cruises a radio receiver for weather forecasts is essential.

Radar reflector: of adequate performance, for cruising in the open sea or in busy shipping channels, or when engaged in sea-angling. Preferably mounted at least ten feet above sea level.

Engine Tool Kit, handbook and spare parts.

Spare engine: even small power craft should have a small extra outboard motor. It may not be necessary in safe restricted inland waters.

Bosun's bag: containing whipping twine, seizing wire, shackles, bulldog clips, canvas, palm and needles, knife, marlin spike and other goodies to personal choice. Not needed for power boats unless used for activities with the students.

Fire extinguisher: where fuel is carried, at least one fire extinguisher of not less than 3 lb (1.5 kg) capacity, dry powder should be fitted. If there is also a galley, then there ought to be two extinguishers.

Boarding ladder: for vessels with a high freeboard, a fixed or folding ladder saves strain on the crew. Many handicapped and overweight people experience great difficulty in boarding, especially from the water. So 'high freeboard' must be interpreted very flexibly.

Fog horn: aerosol horns are useful if used frequently, but the nozzle easily becomes clogged with salt from sea air. Trumpet-type horns seem to be infallible.

Name, number or sail number: should be painted prominently on the vessel or on dodgers in letters or figures at least nine inches (22cm) high.

Oars or paddles: oars (with rowlocks) are more efficient than paddles.

First Aid Box: to include anti-seasickness tablets.

Bivvy Bag

Sleeping Bag

Maps or Charts

Water-resistant Torch

Tow Rope

Other equipment
It is generally better to avoid gadgets and specialised equipment designed to assist handicapped sailors, unless essential, and aim to utilise standard equipment supplemented by imaginative improvisation, particularly if the boat is on loan. For example, an inconveniently sited tiller could have an extension attachment, or be operated by 'remote control' using improvised rope and pulleys by one helmsman or ropes operated by two helmsmen on either side working together. Grab-handles can be made from ropes, spars or boat hooks.

Ropes (warps) are useful for all manner of things from knotting to keel-hauling.

Physical support for severely handicapped people can be given by a 'vacuum support', a polystyrene filled bag which deflates to fit snugly around or under the body. Available from

Innovention (vacuum support) Products Ltd, 51, Coldharbour Lane, Bushey, Hertfordshire, ND2 3NU.

Portable folding chairs or stools can be useful supplements to static seating which is often inconveniently placed for people for whom stretching is difficult. The chairs may need to be tied in place. Of course, such chairs may prove more trouble than they are worth, and after the skipper has been pinioned to the duckboards a few times by a recalcitrant chair he may abandon it on a passing buoy. But do experiment!

Safety considerations

When sailing in flotilla conditions, unless all the boats are unquestionably seaworthy and able to assist each other, the fleet would ideally be accompanied by an escort and a rescue craft. The escort craft would be a substantial launch sufficiently powerful to tow all craft in any anticipated sea conditions, and be large enough to accommodate all crews. The rescue craft needs to be fast, highly manoeuvrable, and stable when stationary. Dories and semi-inflatables are the most popular craft for this role. The propeller must have an effective guard. The advantage of the semi-inflatable over the dory is that its flexible cushions prevent damage to equipment or bodies, enabling it to work safely at close quarters. Speed is essential for transferring patients quickly to the facilities of the escort craft or the shore. It is impossible to dictate a set ratio of safety craft to instructional craft, as so much will depend on the sailing location, weather and water conditions. Also, for most organisations and individuals a compromise has to be reached to balance the desire to provide sailing experiences and ideal safety measures, with available resources.

Local weather and, where appropriate, sea conditions, should be checked beforehand. Information can be obtained from Coastguard stations, RAF stations, local and national radio and television.

The two serious dangers most likely to confront the sailor are drowning and hypothermia. Staff can do a lot to minimise the dangers.

Drowning: if possible see every member of the sailing group in the water beforehand, wearing lifejackets and normal aids such as calipers. Water confidence is essential for small dinghies, but need not be for larger craft. An ability to swim should be considered desirable. If immersion is unavoidable, staff must keep students calm, reassured and cheerful, before, during and after the experience. Capsize practice in safe controlled conditions is the only certain way of preventing panic during an uncontrolled capsize. For the novice sailor the only thing more alarming than an unexpected, unprepared-for capsize, is the sight of his instructor abandoning ship. (Instructors please note.) All staff should be conversant with resuscitation techniques.

Hypothermia: this condition develops when the body temperature falls below about 35°C (95°F). Hypothermia is commonly caused by immersion in cold water; inadequate protection against a cold environment, particularly if the casualty is exhausted or wearing wet clothes; or simply from general exposure to cold. The ability of the body to protect itself from the cold is lessened by drugs, certain medical conditions such as diabetes, and an individual's poor physical condition. All physically handicapped people must be considered to be particularly at risk. The early stages of hypothermia are often referred to in laymen's terms as 'exposure'. Symptoms include: irrational behaviour, complaints of coldness and tiredness, physical and mental lethargy, abnormality of vision, slurred speech, shivering fits, sudden outbursts of energy or violent language, muscle cramp, extreme pallor and occasionally a fainting fit. Not all of these symptoms may be present, nor necessarily in this order.

Immersion in cold water (i.e. below 15°C) causes severe chilling and may result in hypothermia, even if immersion is not prolonged. The temperature of British coastal water, even in summer, rarely rises above 15°C. If prolonged immersion is anticipated, to reduce heat loss, remain motionless, keep the head and face clear of the water with the arms and legs close to the body, and wear a hat. Anyone who is immersed, for however short a time, must be treated for exposure.

Methods of treatment will vary according to condition, the equipment immediately available, and the severity of the exposure. The earlier treatment is given, the less extreme it needs to be. If exposure is mild, the addition of hat, gloves, extra sweater and windproof anorak may suffice. More severe exposure may necessitate removing the patient's wet clothing and putting him into a sleeping bag. A fit companion can go into the sleeping bag alongside him to give bodily warmth. A bivvy bag is pulled around the sleeping bag. Provide shelter, food with high sugar content, and warm sweet drinks. Be alert in extreme cases for respiratory failure and failure of the heart (no pulse, blue lips, dilated pupils). But check very carefully, for a casualty with hypothermia may have a very slow heartbeat which is difficult to detect, and an imperceptible breathing rate. The patient should, as soon as possible, be placed in a pre-warmed bed in a warm room. The casualty should be medically examined as soon as possible if exposure (hypothermia) is suspected.

Exposure and hypothermia are much easier to prevent than to treat. Warm sensible clothing is essential, and all staff must be constantly vigilant for signs and symptoms in themselves as well as the students. Every effort should be made to keep the feet dry, especially when entering the boat.

Sailing and the teacher
Embarking and disembarking often takes a long time, so should be treated as part of the whole experience.

If a long-term programme can be arranged, then most students can be taught skills and nautical vocabulary – slowly and in small steps.

Try to involve everyone in doing something – steering, drawing sheets, lookout, reefing and so on. In this context, as well as for safety considerations, a ratio of one member of staff to each student can give personal and repeated instructions as required for each individual task. The staff should aim to show and guide rather than impose an excess of factual information: avoid too much, too soon. It is helpful to know the individual students – their extent of hearing and vision, and their level of understanding and accumulated knowledge. This dictates the words, phrases and gestures to be used and the pace of instruction. Avoid sophisticated and frightening techniques and experiences until you know the group. For instance, keep the boat upright, and if a student is helming, sail on a reach to allow a wide margin of steering error. Adventurous experiences are desirable for the students, but the instructor must remain in complete control, putting the craft in apparent danger if he chooses to, but never in real danger.

Generate a feeling of unity and team spirit. One way of encouraging this is for each person to bring something to share (usually edible, such as sweets, nuts or crisps).

Engine controls are often fascinating. Deaf people can usually feel the vibrations of the engine, and visual gestures indicating more or less vibration can be given by the instructor.

Changing seats can help prevent feelings of monotony.

A boat is an ideal means of transport for teaching several aspects of environmental studies: exploring caves, measuring tidal flow and river profiles, taking samples of silt, water, plankton and plants, or historical harbour studies.

The boat is also a stable platform for drawing, painting and mapping. Large aids such as felt boards could be used for orientation, sticking symbols on a map, or building an 'identikit' of the boat.

Soundings can be taken using conventional lead lines or improvised lines with cotton reels or knots to denote measurement. The anchor can be utilised as a teaching aid by raising, lowering, pulling the boat, seeing effect of wind and tide, and so on. A tape recorder can provide a lot of enjoyment, particularly for blind people. A period of quiet can be instructive, with the boat moored, eyes covered, and sounds identified by hearing only.

For a teaching platform, two boats can raft up, leaving one instructor to control the craft, and the other free to concentrate on teaching.

Other integrated activities might include fishing (usually more successful on inland waters), rowing, sailing round obstacle courses, picking up moorings, simulated man overboard drill, changing boats, trying out different types of craft, looking at other vessels, knotting and whipping, weather and bird watching. Most mentally retarded people, and especially children, have a short concentration span, so short sailing or boating trips interspersed with other activities may be most suitable. These other activities could include rock-pooling and beach-combing – looking for anything of interest: shells, artifacts, stones or marine life beneath stones and seaweeds; the staff need not be ecology or biology specialists. A walk to a place of interest, exploring caves on foot, rock traversing, swimming, shopping or indeed anything at all. A picnic never fails to enliven the proceedings.

But for the more adventurous, perhaps living on board may provide the ultimate challenge.

Cruising holidays

There can be few pleasures in life to compare with the realisation that you are in charge of a small part of your universe. Cruising, for those converted to its charms and aware of its dangers, is the only way to travel. Gliding through an iron-grey sea, cutting across waves using the wind and tide to take you from one part to another; no timetables, traffic jams or queues. How pleasant to sail into one of the many thousand small ports available to the cruising sailor. One can sit and watch the elegant heron delicately weaving its way along the shore searching out its supper whilst your own is sending up mouth-watering smells from the galley below! The sense of well-being as you lie in your bunk listening to the clinking of the halyards against the mast and the gentle lapping of blue water against the hull can, for the dedicated cruiser, never be equalled by any land-locked pleasure.

The bonus is that for those handicapped people who are prepared to take the initial steps towards becoming a competent crew member on a cruiser the pleasures are the same. Gone are the clumsy aids needed to move across the land; no wheelchairs or crutches are needed; no specially adapted motor cars. All are replaced by a sleek, elegant boat whose very existence is due to thousands of years of evolution to produce the efficient hull shapes that grace every small harbour in the country.

A rosy picture indeed, but as with all things there are two sides to every story, so perhaps a cautionary tale may well balance the picture. A few years ago I was leading a group of young handicapped student sailors on a routine trip from Fowey to Polperro along the beautiful but dangerous coastline. Before setting off the weather forecast was checked and the meteorological office gave us the good news – clear skies,

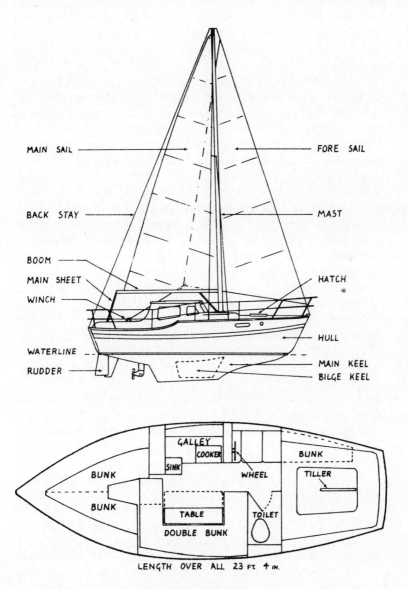

MAIN SAIL — FORE SAIL

BACK STAY — MAST

BOOM — MAIN SHEET — WINCH — HATCH

WATERLINE — HULL

RUDDER — MAIN KEEL — BILGE KEEL

GALLEY — COOKER — BUNK

SINK — WHEEL — TILLER

BUNK

BUNK — TABLE — TOILET

DOUBLE BUNK

LENGTH OVER ALL 23 FT 4 IN.

The motor sailer

moderate winds, good visibility – no problems. The boat was collected from her moorings and we set sail. The voyage went well and work on coastal navigation was proceeding according to plan.

Gradually a group of clouds on the horizon moved nearer and the weather became worse almost by the minute. The wind rose and the boat dug deep into the increasing sea. Spray was now showering everyone on board. It became obvious that the entrance to Polperro was too dangerous for us to attempt and the decision to return to Fowey was made, much to the dismay of my now frightened crew. To their credit they behaved well and their discomfort was made less by the fact that they were all equipped with waterproofs and life jackets. A gentle day's cruise was now turning into a battle between us and the elements! The wind was now almost too much for our already reefed sails, so these were lowered and the engine then took up the strain.

We now depended on that piece of boat equipment that sailing sailors often despise – the engine. Had that engine failed we could have been swept onto the jagged rocks only a few hundred yards away. Fortunately our equipment is all maintained to a very high standard and soon the familiar landmarks of Fowey came into view. As we passed under St Catherine's Castle the squall ceased and moved away, the sun came out and we were able to reflect on the lessons the sea had taught us. Not one member of that crew dropped out of the course and all have gone on over the years to enjoy many happy cruising adventures. Never take anything at sea for granted. But how can we start?

There are many routes. Unfortunately finance does influence your ambitions. Let us assume that your means are limited. You may be able to consider the purchase of a secondhand craft. A suitable secondhand cruiser will cost between £2,000 and £20,000. If you have a regular income you should be able to raise a marine mortgage. This could cover up to 80% of the cost of the boat and the repayments would be spread over several years. However, the cost of owning the boat is considerable. Mooring fees, fuel, repairs and maintenance will all add up. Unless you live close to your boat and have a great deal of spare time, owning a boat is not a particularly viable proposition. It can be made more practical if you share a boat with three or four other people. This has particular advantages for the beginner if the other members of the syndicate are experienced sailors who are prepared to take a novice under their wing.

If you want to own a boat but cannot afford the price involved you may be tempted to build the craft yourself, again sharing the cost and with several people making this project easier. There are hundreds of kit-boats on the market and these can be bought at various stages of completion. However, when you cost out the boat be sure to check the prices of everything you need to complete it. Half completed boats can often be seen in back gardens because an aspiring sailor has run out of funds halfway through his labours!

For most of us the best alternative is to charter a boat. This is fairly easy to do and involves paying a 'rent' to the boat's owner for the use of the craft over a set period. Charters come in various forms; the basic one is described as 'bare boat' and as the term suggests you just get the boat and you provide all food, water and fuel and assume temporary ownership of the boat. The next is 'skippered charter' where the boat comes together with its skipper, often the owner. This form of chartering is particularly useful for the sailor with limited experience and, provided the skipper is prepared to teach, this is a very good way to learn boat skills. Another very popular way is the 'flotilla charter' where you sail as a member of a fleet of boats following a lead yacht. At least one member of your crew needs to be experienced. This type of chartering has the advantage that most of your fellow charterers will be of similar levels of experience and of course the more willing hands around to lift wheelchairs and their occupants on and off the boats the better! Be warned – the social life on a flotilla holiday is every bit as exacting as the sailing itself. In my opinion flotilla sailing is the best way for handicapped sailors to learn and enjoy cruising. Once the basics have been learnt it is highly likely that you will become confirmed flotilla sailors and every holiday from then on will be taken 'on the water'.

When planning a trip or a week's holiday great attention should be paid to the food required. You should carry enough supplies to last for three days. Basics such as coffee, instant soups, instant meals, chocolate, sugar, tea, etc. It is always a good idea to make up a pile of sandwiches before you sail, since a rolling boat does not provide the ideal environment for producing 'haute cuisine'!

So far we have examined the possibilities available to handicapped sailors using the unmodified equipment available to able-bodied sailors. If, however, you feel that a more specialised introduction to cruising would suit you better, the specially converted craft such as *Sparkle* and *The Lord Nelson*, mentioned earlier in this chapter, are available to you.

Cruising the coastline of Cornwall for me is the best form of boating available; however, I would be the first to understand that initially the disabled person may well feel a little daunted by the prospect of a life on the ocean wave. An attractive alternative could well be found on the many hundreds of miles of canals that thread their way through much of Great Britain. Ever since the Industrial Revolution and the golden age of canals, these inland waterways have provided a peaceful escape into the countryside. Several of the canals now have narrow boats especially adapted to the needs of wheelchair users. The Peter Le Marchant Trust, for example, is able to provide day trips and longer holidays on two well equipped 70 foot long narrow boats. Canal cruising would be ideal for the family and a more relaxing form of travelling would be hard to imagine. Further information on canals and canal holidays is available in the book *Out of Doors with Handicapped People*.

Cruising, then, is a contagious disease which once contracted you will find hard to relinquish. Who knows, in a few years from now, you could be cruising the Florida Keys or dropping anchor off some small whitewashed Greek fishing village.

3 Just paddling about

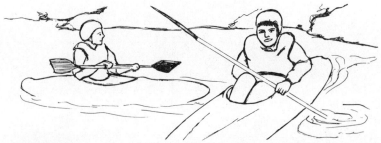

Introduction

Paddling lazily down the river, entering the swirling white
waters of small rapids or toying with the gentle swell and waves
along the coastline – canoeing is perhaps the most challenging
adventure for the disabled person on water. Once in the canoe
you are on your own, and while there may be many others
around you, they cannot help you stabilise your craft or
prevent a capsize.

Canoeing is a great boost to one's confidence, but it needs to
be approached with caution and introduced slowly to the
handicapped beginner. The sight of large open expanses of
rough water will do nothing to develop that confidence in the
mind of a young mentally retarded adolescent or of someone
who has spent his or her whole life in a wheelchair. Rather the
warm, still water of a swimming pool is the place to begin,
ideally in a craft that has good stability.

There are many designs of canoe: most of us are best
acquainted with the *kayak*, developed from the hunting craft of
the Eskimo, made originally from animal skins and moved
with a double-bladed paddle. Modern kayaks are constructed
from glass fibre, giving strength, being relatively maintenance-
free but if necessary easy to repair. The type of kayak used
initially may depend on availability but should be selected for
stability rather than speed, and will therefore be shorter in
length and broader in the beam than sporty models.

Many people working with disabled canoeists have found
great success with the *Caranoe*. Originally designed as a 'fun
canoe' for family holidays on the river, lake or sea it was
quickly seen to be an ideal shape for safely introducing this
adventure to handicapped participants. The short length

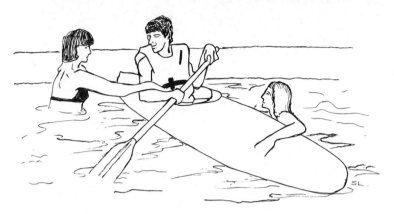

The Caranoe – ideal for pool canoeing

enables it to be used conveniently in a swimming pool; the broad flat beam makes it stable even when the occupant leans heavily to one side or perhaps makes erratic movements, and the large cockpit facilitates easy entry – or exit! This latter feature is especially important when one considers the body shape of many physically disabled people or the fact that legs may not bend or straighten easily. The mentally retarded person is quite often considerably overweight and the Caranoe is an ideal design for their use. An additional feature is the adaptability for fixing a back-support which converts the pre-shaped seat into a far more comfortable resting structure, ideal for those with limited body posture.

Recently three more moulded fibre canoes have been designed, essentially as fun craft but with great potential for use by handicapped canoeists under safe conditions. In this respect they are an ideal way to introduce the activity to those who may never feel the excitement of sitting on the water in a small craft. The *Duette, Kadet* and *Kayetta* are all produced by Hotelcraft Ltd and were designed by Jonathan Spragg. They are highly stable and have non-trap cockpits. We found the Kayetta to be robust in construction, the deep draught giving good directional stability. Turning the craft was surprisingly easy. The large cockpit allowed us to fit any shape of body into the craft, using blocks of polystyrene to give support in the best paddling position. Its use in the pool helped individuals gain

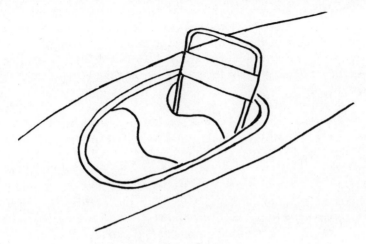

Backrest for a Caranoe

water confidence and certainly have fun! The canoe is suitable for sheltered waters – a lake or river, but the paddler will soon get wet with the very open cockpit in any exposed conditions. However, it stays afloat even when full of water and can support considerable weight, so that both an instructor and a small trainee can sit in the craft together – a very useful way of teaching the mentally handicapped person how to use paddles.

In the pool
Once in the pool it is desirable that the individuals to be introduced to canoeing should first demonstrate their confidence in water. This may be simply by 'play' situations; jumping on the spot while in the water, with occasional squats so that the head is also submerged; standing still and placing the face beneath the water surface; floating on the back with an instructor giving support at the head and shoulders. Many authorities believe the handicapped canoeist should be able to swim, in the conventional sense, a definite distance. The British Canoe Union recommend a minimum 50 metre standard for most canoeists, but for the disabled person they recognise that this may not be possible. In this case they consider that it is sufficient in group canoeing that the individual should be able to float with confidence after capsizing and coming safely out

of the canoe. However, extra supervision should be provided to preserve a reasonable standard of safety. Clearly lifejackets or buoyancy aids will give greater confidence in the mind of the beginner and provide an additional safety standard. The instructor will also help depending on how he approaches the new pupil.

Communication is all-important: the instructor can either quickly reassure the beginner or destroy his confidence for evermore. Progress by small steps is required and stages should not be rushed. Rather the handicapped canoeist should learn through fun, discovering many things for himself rather than having to be told everything by the instructor. Positioning, balance, paddling, turning will all come eventually to the beginner providing the atmosphere created is conducive to learning. For the mentally handicapped person it is important to avoid confusion in words; demonstration will produce better results than talk. That is not to say that words of encouragement should be forgotten, and it is often possible to talk someone through a difficult patch. During this early routine the instructor should be in the water with his beginner, maintaining eye contact as much as possible. Communication is not only by word of mouth – eyes and facial expression are just as significant.

In the early stages, the canoeist will enter the craft with help from the poolside, with other helpers holding the canoe steady in the water. At this point a paddle is unnecessary and the beginner can use his own hands to paddle around, sensing his own proximity to the water and beginning to feel at home in this new environment. With the more profoundly, multiply-handicapped individual this may be all that is ever achieved – but it is still an adventure for the mentally retarded, cerebral palsied patient from institutional care. Progress will vary between individuals – some may soon be holding their paddle, and mastering the 'feathered' blade. For others it may be desirable to introduce a paddle with both blades facing in the same plane, until the correct wrist action is learned by the new pupil.

An ability to canoe across the pool in a straight line is the initial aim. This can be followed by turning to right and to left, both by paddling more strongly on one side and by holding the

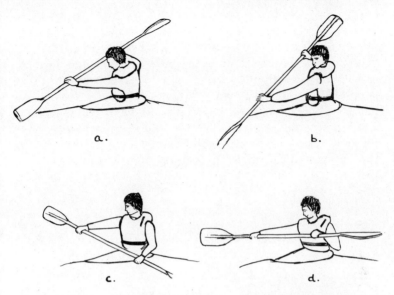

Basic forward paddling strokes using feathered blades

blade in the water, slightly behind the canoeist, and reverse paddling. Finally, the trainee can approach full reverse paddling, looking behind his canoe as he moves backward across the pool. Mastering these basic strokes may well take many lessons, although the bright physically disabled canoeist may learn all of these stages in a single lesson.

A full capsize drill should not be attempted until confidence and enthusiasm have developed, and most instructors would require that canoeists going onto open water should be able satisfactorily to complete such a capsize. In the event of this not being possible the canoeist may be able to accompany the instructor in a double canoe, providing water confidence has been demonstrated. The canoeist who cannot accomplish a correct capsize drill, or who is highly suspect in his efforts, can still safely use one of the 'open' canoes, such as the Duette, Kadet or Kayetta, which have non-trap cockpits. They are quite capable of being used on open waters, although one might get very wet. In the pool the Kayetta is highly suitable, with no danger of the canoeist being trapped when the craft inverts.

The capsize drill should be undertaken in water deep enough

to allow the canoeist to leave the craft when underwater, without fear of hitting his head on the bottom. Ideally the paddle is held in the normal position, but early efforts to capsize might be tried without the paddle. The trainee must roll gently sideways into the water, retaining his seat until the canoe is completely upside down. He releases the paddle, puts his hands on the side of the canoe behind him and keeping his legs straight and still, he leans forward and slides carefully out of the canoe. He is assisted in his actions by gravity and slips from the submerged canoe rather than trying to climb out.

Very often the mentally retarded or physically disabled

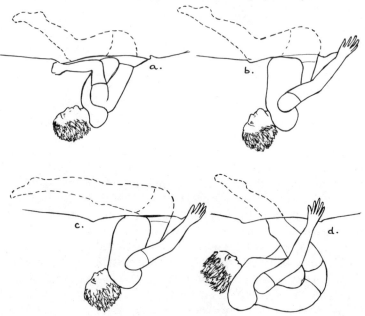

The capsize drill

canoeist will leave the capsizing craft before it completes its turn and is fully upside-down in the water. In this event praise should still be given, although he should be encouraged to repeat the action several times, perhaps as a demonstration to others watching from the pool side. Eventually the correct procedure may develop, but if not this should not preclude the trainee from going onto open water, provided confidence is still maintained. He should be taught to maintain contact with the floating craft, since air trapped inside helps it to float. This cannot be relied upon, however, since movement displaces the air with water and the canoe will gradually sink. Consequently the importance of buoyancy inside the canoe should be stressed, since only this will keep it afloat. No attempt should be made to upright the canoe or to empty the water; rather should the canoeist move along the canoe length towards one end but always keeping in contact. If possible he should regain the paddle but await assistance from the instructor and other helpers. In white water and at sea a spray deck might be necessary to cover the cockpit and stop excess water entering the craft, but this should not be fitted during early capsize drills and is unnecessary on open water in still conditions. Simplicity should be the aim whenever possible.

Much success has been obtained by Ron Moore, Headteacher at a Plymouth Special School, with handicapped young canoeists of wide-ranging disabilities; his personal notes on canoeing with the mentally handicapped, and the chapter he has provided in the BCU *Canoeing Handbook*, have provided a basis for this section. In addition we have gathered a good deal of information and techniques while introducing canoeing to severely handicapped children and adults attending our own basic courses at Churchtown Farm Centre in Cornwall.

For anyone planning a course of canoe instruction, winter can be an ideal time to begin, provided that a heated indoor pool is available. The local recreation centre is the most obvious place to choose, but many special schools and other similar establishments may provide this facility. If an open-air pool is the only available site then it is important to wait until water temperature is high enough to avoid frightening situations in the event of a capsize. Remember that muscles relax in the warmth of the indoor pool but equally become tense in contact with colder waters. Confidence in these colder waters should be demonstrated before the canoe beginner leaves the pool behind for the open river or lake.

The open water scene

Where shall we go, what shall we wear? Who can we take, who will instruct? Many questions continue to arise, even after the initial pool drills. There are safe open-waters but, equally, all water can be dangerous. One should always treat the river, lake, reservoir, canal and sea with care and respect. Where you canoe will often depend on where you live, but initially the water requires to be still or to have as little movement as possible, not to be too deep and preferably to be as confined by banks or shoreline as possible. The scene will be less frightening if the canoeist can maintain eye contact with fixed positions on land. Many towns and cities have a disused canal, park lake or river which may well be ideal for the beginner, but regard should be taken of the nature of the bottom material, since mud and silt can be more dangerous than the water. Ideally select a good sand or gravel bed, free of large rocks and other obstacles and with a water depth of about one metre or slightly more.

A firm bank, landing stage, path or similar hard-standing is necessary for loading into canoes, especially when disabled people are leaving wheelchairs or use hand/arm crutches. The canoe is held at both ends by helpers while the canoeist enters

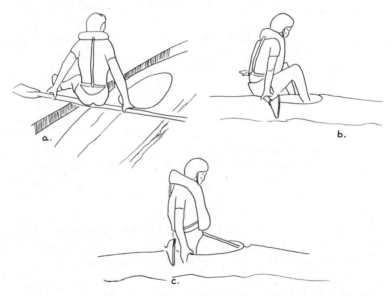

Entering the canoe – using the paddle as a brace for support

the cockpit, often with assistance, or is lifted from the wheelchair and placed in the canoe seat. In this event the wheelchair should be positioned alongside the canoe with the side arm-rest removed. The canoeist can then more easily transfer from chair to canoe. Many disabled young canoeists use wheelchairs on land but can be free of them once on the water and assume the 'normality' of the able-bodied person. Any handicapped person can therefore try this adventure activity provided that all preliminary stages have been undertaken first.

Clearly people will react differently to a situation in open water than when in the pool and this must be taken into consideration before allowing them to proceed. Epilepsy should not preclude someone from canoeing, although it is usually thought that seizures should be under control, and more time might be necessary in the pool stages and in demonstrating cold water safety. In the event of a seizure during a capsize the lifejacket would tend to keep the canoeist pressed up under the canoe and drowning would be probable. The question of *Water Sports and Epilepsy* is the subject of a leaflet published by the Sports Council and the subject is well discussed by Norman Croucher in his book *Outdoor Pursuits for Disabled People*.

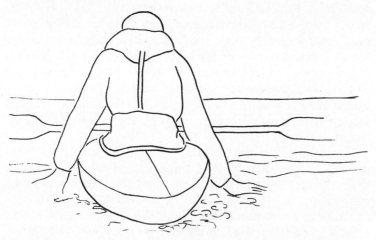

Launching the canoe from a beach or muddy river bank

Open water canoeing, as in the pool, should be taken by slow stages, since most physical handicaps are exaggerated by fatigue and often lead to sensory loss in various parts of the body. Consequently injury to the legs may result when entering the canoe, and pressure sores can develop from sitting still on a hard seat against a hard edge to the cockpit. Cold and impaired circulation will also play a significant role in making the disabled canoeist uncomfortable and tired and may lead to a potentially dangerous situation. Some stress situations can be relieved in advance by ensuring the cockpit is smooth at the edges, providing foam padding, checking inside the canoe for roughness to the legs, providing a back rest and ensuring suitable clothing is worn. While in the pool it might be enough to wear trunks or a swimming costume, but once on open water (even on a hot day) the canoeist requires protection. Wet suits might be ideal, but it is unlikely that many disabled canoeists will possess them, and swimwear worn beneath a sweat shirt or thin jumper, with trousers, rather than jeans, to cover the legs, will be equally suitable.

An approved make of life jacket or buoyancy aid is essential at all times for both trainee canoeists and instructors. Safety helmets may be worn if available, and are important for epileptics, those with brain-damage and certain other physical disabilities. Plimsolls are best on the feet, with thick socks if the feet are sensitive to abrasions or cold. Protection from wind, rain and cold will be achieved by a sweater, cagoule, woollen hat and even gloves, although if it is this cold it is doubtful if the handicapped canoeist should be out on open water. Woollen clothing will tend to trap the water but body heat soon warms this to provide an insulation layer next to the skin, especially if further water movement is reduced by outer clothes – anorak, overtrousers, etc.

Conditions do deteriorate rapidly, however, and the instructors may carry extra clothing in large polythene bags for their trainees. Hot drinks, chocolate and other safety and survival materials should also be carried in the instructor's canoe or in a separate safety craft if this is available. A rubber inflatable dinghy makes an ideal safety boat, with two helpers aboard: one to man the outboard motor and helm the boat, while the other assists the disabled person in the event of a

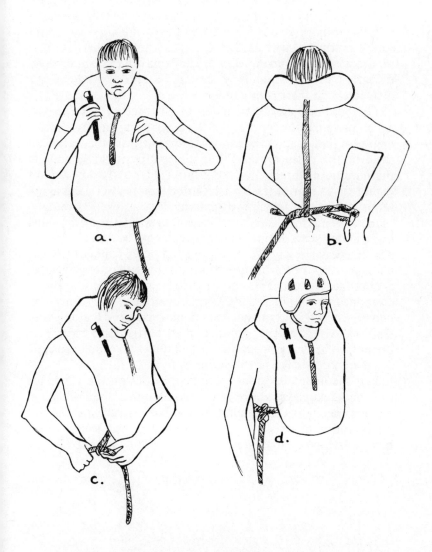

Fitting an approved lifejacket or buoyancy aid and safety helmet

capsize. The safety boat can carry emergency rations, hot drinks in thermos flasks, spare clothing and a sleeping bag in polythene bags; first aid kit, ropes to tow a canoe and extra safety features, such as flares, if sea canoeing is likely. A separate craft is often unnecessary and unavailable but survival resources are not and they should be taken along by the instructors in their own canoes.

The number and experience of instructors and helpers accompanying the group will also vary depending on the degree of handicap of the canoeists, the nature of the water and the total size of the group. While some authorities recommend the minimum standard of the group leader should be that of Senior Instructor of the British Canoe Union (BCU) this again might be difficult to achieve for some organisations wishing to plan canoeing for disabled trainees. Certainly the leader must have many years' canoe experience, know the group and be able to effect a rescue. Being a good individual canoeist will not necessarily make for being a good, safe instructor of a disabled group, but the leader should be encouraged to attend training courses and obtain the BCU qualifications. Assistants and helpers should also include experienced canoeists, along with staff who know the handicapped participants wherever possible. They may not canoe so well but will be indispensable for their knowledge of the trainees.

It is recommended that there be a helper on the water for each handicapped canoeist, who stays alongside that individual and accepts individual responsibility. The instructor should be additional to the basic requirement since he will need to move between trainees to teach techniques. Staff should also be

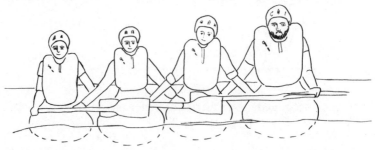

Rafting up – a safe means of keeping young trainees together

available on land to watch the whole group scene and make the group aware of any impending dangers such as a weir, approaching vessel, fallen tree or heavy current. Attention is best attracted by a blown whistle signal and perhaps a red flag, if deaf persons are involved. Blind or partially sighted canoeists can find direction by means of bells or bleepers along the banks of a canal or river, or along the seashore. Transistor radios have been used very successfully as sound signals in this manner, placed at a suitable distance apart on either bank. However, this may not be necessary and a helper paddling behind giving occasional directions may be quite enough help for the blind person.

The trainee may require to be towed by an instructor if he cannot master paddling or is reticent to do so. I have seen a young autistic boy towed in such a manner for half an hour before he decided to take part in the proceedings, picking up his own paddle and beginning to copy his instructor who had towed him for so long. The child ultimately completed the journey under his own steam and was a very different boy from the one who began that day. As he left he was laughing and waving goodbye, very confident of his abilities in a canoe.

Normality should be the aim wherever possible and most handicapped trainees should manage well in a conventional canoe or in the Caranoe. The latter can be fitted with a spray deck, attached by velcro strips, as well as a back rest. In addition the Duette, with its open cockpit, is roomy and very stable and suitable for introducing canoeing to a disabled person. Towing canoes, singles and doubles, are also a convenient means of taking more severely disabled trainees onto open water, thus giving the desirable adventure experience.

Paddle adaptations may be necessary for canoeists who are only capable of using a single arm or where one arm is much stronger. A single paddle design has been tested under the extreme conditions of an expedition of young disabled canoeists to the white river waters of the Dordogne Valley in France. The paddle fits loosely about the arm and the canoe is moved by paddling on alternate sides. Velcro strips can also be used to fix a paddle to mitts worn by the trainee with a weak grip. Often unfeathered paddle blades will help blind canoeists, those with a weak grip or the mentally retarded trainee.

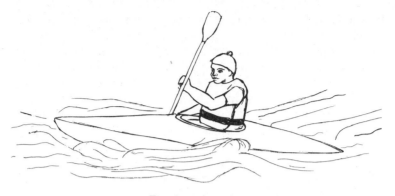

The kayak at sea

Canoe adventure

Once the basic skills have been learnt, a canoe provides numerous opportunities for touring, camping and adventure. In many ways it is an ideal means of transport for the handicapped person, giving a great sense of normality and independence. The wheelchair can be left behind and there are no tiring legs for the walker who must use arm crutches or finds difficulty on land. Clearly there are many plans to be made, not least how to get those very wheelchairs to the site of the camp at the end of the day's travels. Small group canoe camps with mentally retarded young people will provide everyone – staff and handicapped – with a real challenge, but will give great satisfaction when completed. By careful consideration of canoe types it is possible to take the less accomplished canoeist on the tour, although all preliminary stages described for pool and open water canoeing should first be tackled.

The kayak may not be the most suitable design of craft for touring. Open Canadian canoes are in many ways ideal for this form of adventure although are not so readily available in this country as in North America. Touring canoes are, however, more easily located, and both singles and doubles can be constructed for yourselves from glass fibre. A double canoe allows for someone to be taken aboard by the instructor when too tired for solo paddling or after a capsize. The instructor will usually sit behind the trainee where he can watch the behaviour of a mentally retarded individual or see other problems as they arise. Touring canoes are broad in the beam, providing lateral stability but sluggish directional movements. Tourers are bulky and heavy but have ample room to pack equipment for the camp. The handicapped person who is still more at home in the Caranoe should be allowed this craft for touring.

The Canadian canoe has developed from early 'dug-outs' and the Indian birch bark canoe. They were large, working craft carrying heavy, bulky loads for long distances along rivers and providing an essential form of transport in wild country. Modern 'Canadians' are built from aluminium (looking more like large floating bath-tubs), glass fibre and other resilient materials. The canoe is moved by a single bladed paddle and longer models (over 6m) can easily take four persons, each paddling on alternate sides. There is a great deal of freeboard, or height of exposed canoe above the water-line, and a keel running mid-line along the length of the canoe, beneath the water, provides added stability and helps the craft trace a straight line in the water. Seats or thwarts run across the beam, although paddling is often in the kneeling position.

The single-bladed paddle should be of the correct length for the individual, ie. the length should be equal to his height from eye-level to floor in the standing position. One hand is placed at the tip of the shaft in a gripping position, while the other conveniently holds the shaft not too far above the water surface. Thus, a stroke can be effected. Successful movement depends on the crew working as a team and in this respect gives excellent training for mentally handicapped individuals.

The planning of a canoe tour should be as careful as when preparing for a hike in the mountains. Firstly, the distance travelled must be well within the capabilities of the weakest canoeist in the group. If the tour is to be along a river, start upstream and use the natural flow, or in tidal waters such as an estuary travel with the tide and notice the time of tidal change. When at sea move along the edge of the coast, maintaining close contact with the shore at all times and again note tides, wind direction and wave strength. Currents will be an added problem on many open waters. Look at the map and make a preliminary visit to see for yourself the route you are planning to take.

Group size is important, especially when canoe camping,

since this will determine the amount of equipment required. Again make progress in small stages. Initially make a day tour, returning to the same place, with the tide if possible, or arrange for a vehicle to meet you at the other end of the journey. Gradually extend your distance travelled and plan a night in camp at some convenient site to hand. Obtain permission, check that drinking water is available and that the camp area is sheltered and above flood or tidal levels. Toilet facilities may require arranging if you plan to take physically disabled canoeists, and remote camp sites may not be convenient even if attractive propositions. Arrange to arrive at the proposed site at least three hours before dark, to allow sufficient time to erect tents, cook an evening meal and generally get ready for the night.

Packing for a canoe camp is perhaps easier than for hiking and cycling, since the canoe becomes a large rucksack which is paddled rather than carried. Balance the weight evenly throughout the canoe length, with a tendency to stow more at the stern or rear. Load the canoe in the water or at least at the water's edge, as carrying a loaded canoe will often lead to undue stress and even fracture of the canoe body. All items must be enclosed in waterproof polythene bags, or polythene containers. To prevent tearing of bags they can be stored in a canvas kitbag, a travel zip-bag or even a heavy duty plastic sack such as are used for agricultural purposes. Pack the canoe tightly and secure each separate bag inside the body of the craft with fine nylon rope attached to the rear of the seat or to specially inserted fixing points 'welded' in position by glass fibre resin. Remember that a fully loaded canoe may need extra buoyancy, supplied by polystyrene foam blocks or commercially available chemical preparations. Inflatable buoyancy bags or inflated inner tubes can also be used and will fill gaps between luggage. Much of the equipment to be taken will be the same as when planning short hikes and cycle tours (see chapter 6). A spare change of dry clothes is essential and, together with the sleeping bag, must be kept dry at all times, even in the event of a capsize. Lightweight hike tents are most convenient, but if physically disabled canoeists find difficulty in entering a small tent, arrangements will need to be made to deliver a larger frame tent, together with any wheelchairs, by road or by a larger boat. Dehydrated foods are compact and light in weight, and varied meals can be prepared from commercially available brands. A camping gas cooking stove is most convenient for short camps. First aid kit, rubber-encased torch, maps, compass and tow ropes are also essential equipment. Finally, remember to pack last the items you will need first. It is frustrating to need a plaster for your blistered hand only to find it was nearest to the end point of your canoe.

Rather than undertake day-camps by canoe it may be easier to plan a permanent canoe camp for a weekend or a full week. Considerations will be similar to any other camping programme (see chapter 7) except that access to good canoeing water is essential. A lakeside or river may be most suitable; excellent camps have been arranged for several years on several sites along the River Tamar. Here there is a great sense of both fun and adventure amongst the handicapped canoe campers who are well integrated with experienced able-bodied canoeists and instructors. Each camp lasts a week in July and again progress is made by gentle successive stages. Not all canoeists will have previous experience and many learn their techniques on open water. A rubber inflatable craft acts as a rescue vessel and there is very adequate supervision. Plenty of attention is given to the camp, as well as to the canoeing, so that by the end everyone is able to undertake a lengthy tour down river. Disability is left behind, only to be re-assumed as a vehicle approaches the landing point to deliver wheelchairs to the athletic-looking young canoeists. Observers are usually puzzled and amazed as canoeists stagger from their craft or are pushed away in their wheelchairs!

Perhaps the ultimate canoe adventure will be the excitement of an expedition, either to unusual home waters or to another country. For the disabled paddler this will represent a considerable challenge, probably never to be exceeded in his own lifetime. Most canoeists will never achieve such a goal, but Treloar College has organised canoe travels on French rivers, with handicapped girls disabled by cerebral palsy and spina bifida, and in 1982 a full-scale expedition, 'Kayak France '82', was launched by the Churchtown Farm staff. Linking with French kayakists, the expedition members experienced a truely international flavour to their adventures on the River Ariège in the Midi-Pyrenées. The complete team of sixteen included young people disabled by cerebral palsy, polio, spina bifida and accident trauma, but despite physical limitations all successfully canoed on the varied waters of the region. From Longué, in the Loire, everyone travelled south to train on the Dordogne river, where a French television company filmed the first two days' activities for 'La Porte Ouverte', a weekly programme about people with handicaps. French culture became mixed with adventure – different food, different language, different ways. Important linked activities introduced members of the group to the insects and birds; collections of botanical specimens were made and a survey of the stream life of local waters. Towns and villages yielded new history, new buildings and shops. Education at its very best!

The river proved to be exciting and challenging. The team was able to experience the quieter lower reaches of the Ariège; its fuller bouncier sections at Foix; percolating rocky upper stretches near Ax-les-Thermes as well as subterranean sections in the caves near Foix. Each section of the river was travelled with part or all of the team in kayaks, with an inflatable raft acting as security. The general concensus was that the expedition was an exceptional opportunity to canoe in thrilling water with the security and confidence of experts in kayaking and water safety. It was a unique opportunity for handicapped and able-bodied members together, to extend the limits of their own expectations, not just on the river, but also in their new cultural and social circumstances.

Linked activities
Observing wildlife from a canoe can be a very different experience from being on land and looking out across the river, lake or sea. Birds are seen from close by, nesting among reeds at the water's edge; herons stand still before a rapid dart is made to catch fish or frogs, and a kingfisher might suddenly fly past close to the river banks. A small pair of binoculars can easily accompany the canoeist and be on hand to note each different bird seen or to watch the behaviour of courting and nesting individuals. Perhaps this could be linked with an interest in photography, and often the silence of the canoe will permit a picture to be taken from much nearer than would

otherwise be possible. Even if you do not want to photograph birds, a selection of pictures illustrating your route along the river, interesting buildings or landmarks passed, will do a great deal to enhance your log book, when you come to write up an account of each canoe trip. Keeping such a log is considered important by the various award-giving bodies, such as the British Canoe Union, or the Duke of Edinburgh Award scheme. Incidentally, a canoe journey may well be a good idea for your expedition section at the Bronze, Silver and Gold standards of the Award scheme (see chapter 7).

A canoe is also an adventurous means of exploring the coastline. Enter a sea cave, edge around a stack or between the rocky uprights of an arch. Experience the power of the surf and the movement of waves beneath you. Realise the forces that have carved the shape of our coastline over thousands of years.

At sea, canoeing along the rocky shoreline at low water permits a startling glimpse of an entirely new world – the submarine regions around our coastline. Long filamentous seaweeds are anchored to the rocks by small button-like discs and look rather more like brown-green bootlaces than plants; broad-bladed kelps, complete with brown, leathery, finger-like fronds and a thick tough stalk fixed securely by a root-like holdfast to the rocks – these, and many more marine organisms are a world apart. No views from on land can compare with the sights to be seen from the sea itself and a canoe makes this all very possible since it can approach the rocks with ease and one can paddle above the kelps which are attached in deeper water. Starfish, sea urchins, small shoals of fish, crabs and lobsters are but some of the animals on view, and with modern waterproof cameras such as the Minolta now available, which will take good colour photographs even when submerged below the water surface, a new hobby suddenly becomes possible and that ocean world can be taken home with you – at least on film.

4 At the water's edge

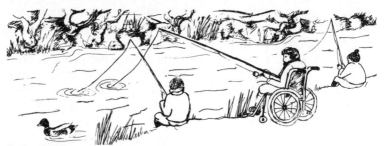

Introduction

Although I am concerned with the promotion of all water based activities for handicapped people I must confess that I am more than a little interested in the sport of angling. Not that I am by any means unique in this; there are more than three million anglers in this country alone and world wide angling is the most popular participant sport of all. In fact it is alleged that there are more anglers than all other sportsmen put together!

It's not all that easy to establish just why so many men and women take up the sport in the first instance, although there are plenty of different explanations why, once having started, so many continue with it: 'it's relaxing'; 'it's exciting'; 'it's a quiet, simple occupation'; 'there's so much to it that it's always interesting', and so on. But what triggers people off in the beginning I just cannot find out. I have a theory that it is something to do with man's hunting instinct coming to the fore.

But what about the safety aspect? Any activity on or near water carries with it a risk factor. Angling is practically the only water based sport that does not carry with it a requirement that all participants must be able to swim or be very confident in cold water, before they take up the sport; the other activities also have the benefit of wearing life jackets or buoyancy aids. To wear these would make some angling impossible. Nevertheless, some provision of safety equipment ought to be included when groups go to the water, and water safety ought to be recognised as an essential part of angling education.

Let us have a closer look at what is involved in the art of angling and see if there might not be something for you in this activity. First of all, the word angler comes from an old Anglo-Saxon word which means a hook or bend, and is just one method of catching fish. All anglers are fishermen – not all fishermen are anglers. Generally the word angler refers to those who fish for pleasure rather than for profit or a living.

The Fish

Sea fish
Not much is needed in the way of explanation when it comes to sea fish. We all know there are fish in the sea and most of us will know a little about some of them, even if it's only from going to the fish and chip shop! What is not generally known is that some species of sea fish come into our rivers and estuaries and travel quite a long way upstream. I have caught small dabs, a flatfish, in the River Thames outside Traitors Gate at the Tower of London.

Game fish
These include the salmon and trout, some of which spend quite a lot of time in the sea but which breed in fresh water. These need clean, fresh, well oxygenated water in which to breed, and so these fish can be found in those waterways which have these qualities. Many reservoirs and manmade lakes have been stocked with trout, mainly rainbow, so that game fishing of one sort or another can be enjoyed all over the country, even in our major cities.

Coarse fish
These include all freshwater fish, other than game fish; they are many and varied. Some, like the barbel, require reasonably clean, unpolluted water which has a gravel bed; others like the carp can tolerate a less clean environment which has a muddy bed.

The three groups of fish live, in a sense, in zones, but these zones overlap so that you might in some circumstances catch at the same spot a sea fish and a coarse fish, while further upstream you might catch a coarse fish or a game fish.

Fish come in a whole range of different shapes and sizes, but the fins and lateral line are common to all. Next time you go by a fishmonger's shop have a look at the fish on display and see if you can pick out the common factors and how they differ from species to species. The range of sizes is quite impressive, ranging from the tiny minnow, weighing only a few grams, to the huge sharks weighing many hundreds of kilos.

There are plenty of books which will enable the prospective angler to find out all the information that he or she might wish to know about fish. A study of the quarry is an essential part of the make-up of the successful angler. The more you know about a fish and its habitat the greater your chance of locating it and catching it. This becomes apparent when you realise that fish, unlike other types of wild life, are not often seen until after they have been caught. I do not believe that fish are particularly intelligent but they are extremely wary and have superb instincts which can make them difficult to catch. For millions of years they have been preyed upon by members of their own family group, other species of fish, reptiles, birds, mammals and of course man, so to survive in spite of being constantly hunted they must have something a little bit special which has prevented them from vanishing forever.

We humans react in an emergency after a very short period of time. The fish reacts immediately. It also has a sense of smell second to none and can detect the smallest amount of any substance, even though it might have been diluted in many hundreds of parts of water; and last but not least it is extremely cautious of anything that appears strange or unusual.

So what can we learn from all this? First of all the fish, through its lateral line, can detect the slightest variation in water pressure and the smallest amount of vibration. Therefore you must avoid all unnecessary movement at the point at which you are fishing. Secondly, you must try and ensure that you do not transfer smells, such as tobacco or soap, which might be on your hands, to the bait you are using and baits must be prepared in as natural a way as possible.

Having now learnt something of the fish and its habitat, we shall have to find a method of angling which will enable us to catch it. That method might, to some degree, depend on the nature of our disability. So let's leave that for a moment and have a look at some of the general equipment we shall all need if we are going to be anglers.

Angling equipment

Hooks: one of the first items of equipment made by man for the catching of fish. Stone-age man used hooks made from bone and today everyone knows what a hook looks like. However, what most people do not know is that hooks come in a huge

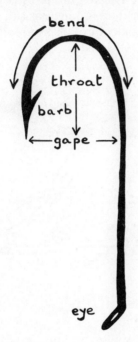

The basic pattern of the hook

range of sizes, shapes and, to a lesser degree, colours. You might be surprised to see how many parts there are to a simple thing like a hook. Whatever type or size of hooks you decide to use, make sure that you buy the best you can afford – cheap hooks have a nasty habit of straightening out or breaking.

Line: most line used today is made from nylon, but once again it comes in different sizes and colours. The size of the line – its thickness, not its length – is dictated by its breaking strain, and that is how one buys it: one hundred yards of 1 kilo (2 lb) line or one hundred yards of 9 kilo (20 lb) line. The breaking strain is intended to indicate the limit to which a line can be stretched before it will break. However, in actual fishing the breaking strain is much lower, as any knots that are used, such as tying the line to the hook, can considerably reduce the strength of the line. The different colour of line is, in my opinion, one of personal preference. The amount of line one requires depends on the type of fishing one is doing. Basically one only needs line and hook to be an angler but this is only allowed in sea fishing.

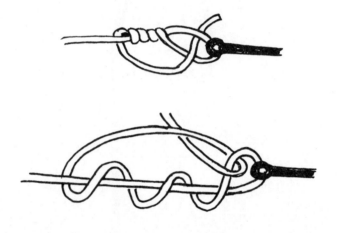

Hook knots

The use of a rod is mandatory in both coarse and game fishing; in the latter it becomes a little more complicated as the type of line is completely different from that used in coarse and sea fishing. Most game fishing is by use of an imitation fly and the line has to be fairly heavy in order to get enough weight to cast. Some game lines are required to float; others to sink either slowly or fast.

Rods: again these come in various types and are made for specific types of fishing and specific methods. The right rod for the type of fishing you intend to follow is essential. In most cases one should always get as large a rod as one can manage. Avoid buying boys' rods, or those kits which are supposed to contain all the gear one wants to go coarse or sea fishing.

Apart from being obligatory, the rod is a useful tool. It helps one to fish over different kinds of obstructions, such as reeds or rocks, to be found at the water's edge; it enables one to fish over very shallow water to reach a reasonable depth; it also acts as an extension of the arms and in so doing helps you to control a hooked fish over a greater area; and lastly it acts as a shock absorber. Remember about the fish reacting much faster than we do? Well the sudden movements of the fish are taken up by the rod tip and without this there would be many occasions when sudden movements of the fish could break the line if one did not have a rod to act in the way it does. With rods one always has a reel; nevertheless one can fish without a reel by using not a rod but a pole.

Pole: basically a pole is a rod without the rings which guide the line from the reel to the rod tip or the reel fittings. Line is fixed to the tip of the pole and should be no shorter than the length of pole that you can manage in one piece. Poles are sometimes telescopic, or come to pieces in sections. They can be as little as $2\frac{1}{2}$m (8 ft) long or in excess of 8m (25 ft). You should always get a pole which is as long as you can comfortably use. Pole fishing has distinct advantages and is used a lot in modern day competitive fishing. However, poles do restrict the different methods of angling that are available to the angler who uses a rod and reel.

Reel: we have three main types of reel. Not, as one might think, for the three different sections of the sport, but for various methods. There are within the three types many variations, some of which would suit particular disabilities better than others. What might suit some individuals might not suit others and a little care needs to be taken when selecting one. The very first type of reel that man used was the *centre pin reel*, and it is still used today, mostly for game fishing, although examples can be seen in both sea and coarse angling. The centre pin is simply a spool which revolves around a centre pin.

The second type is the *fixed spool reel* which, unlike the centre pin, is fixed on the rod at right angles; as its name implies it does not move but relies on a pick-up device to wind spare line onto the spool. Casting is achieved by pushing the pickup to one side, which will allow the line to fall off in coils. This is perhaps the most popular type of fishing reel, being used for all types of fishing.

The third type of reel is the *multiplier* which works on the same principle as the centre pin but is much broader and has gears enabling the spool to revolve three or more times to one revolution of the handle. Mostly it is used for sea fishing, when much more line is used than is normal in other types of fishing.

Most of the latter two reels have a device which can be adjusted to the breaking strain of the line that you are using. This means that as the pull on the line approaches the point at which the line might break, the spool starts to slip, letting line off automatically.

Floats: these are used mainly in coarse fishing but are sometimes used in sea fishing and, where permitted, on some trout waters. The float is simply a device to suspend a bait in the water at the required depth, and it acts as a visual indicator

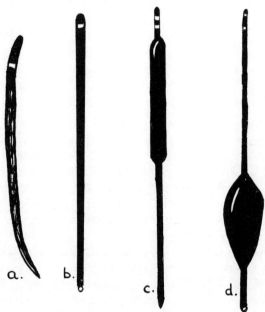

Floats: a) quill;   b) stick;   c) balsa/cane stick;   d) waggler stick

of a bite taking place. Because most floats require lead shot, to cock them, the weight involved also makes casting much easier. Floats are used in fast, slow or still waters and there are hundreds of different types. The right float for the right circumstances makes fishing much more positive and reliable, and this is a subject that one needs to study in some depth to maximise one's results.

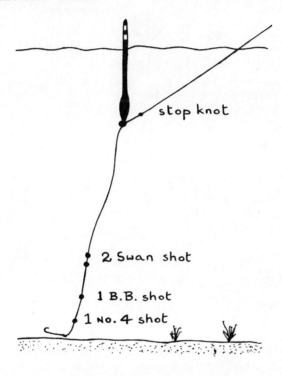

Slider float showing shotting

Shots: these are not only used to cock, or balance, the floats but also have other purposes. The shot comes in different sizes and is in fact the same as is used in shotgun cartridges. The only difference is that the angler's shot has a slit in it and should be made of soft lead. The split shot, if made of hard lead, can damage the line and it's not uncommon for breaks to occur at points where split shot has been pressed too hard on the line.

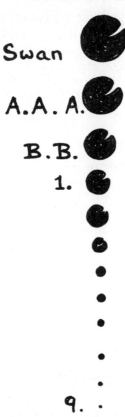

Swan

A.A.A.

B.B.

1.

9.

Size range of split shot

Ledgers: ledgering is a method of fishing without a float and is used exclusively for fishing on the river or sea bed. It is probably the most popular method for sea anglers although it has benefits when applied to coarse fishing. Ledgers are different types and shapes of lead weights through which the line passes freely. Lead split shot is used as a stopper to prevent the ledger moving too close to the hook.

Lures and spinners: these are usually artificial imitations of various forms of aquatic life on which fish might feed. They are made of various materials and the method requires that they be cast out into the water and then retrieved by winding in the line.

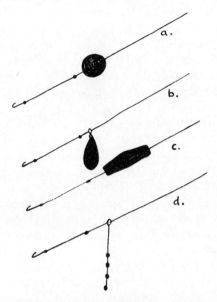

Ledger weights: a) drilled bullet;   b) arsley bomb;
c) sliding coffin;   d) swan shots

Lures glide and wobble through the water while spinners, as
one might expect, spin or revolve. One can, under lures, include
the flies used by the game angler, although this is a subject in its
own right. Also, the fly is not always retrieved – in dry fly-
fishing for example the fly is allowed to remain stationary on
the water.

Bits and pieces: there are many other items of equipment, some
of which are aids and some of which are essentials. You will
require a small pair of scissors or nail clippers to cut line and
trim up the knots, and a disgorger to remove hooks from the
fish without damaging them, since in coarse fishing all fish
should be returned to the water as soon as possible. In both
game and sea fishing one is only allowed to retain fish over a
certain size and in game itself there may be limitations on the
number of fish one is allowed to remove from the water. To
help conserve the fish a cloth is of benefit when handling them
but some may suggest that wet hands are better than a cloth.
Fish are covered with a protective layer of slime-like substance

– the use of thick dry cloths can remove this. I always use a thin but large cotton cloth which is wetted at the water's edge. A landing net is also required and, when taking part in a competition, a keep net. Both of these items are subject to regulations; the nets on both must be made from knotless material and should be as long as one can afford.

Baits: sea fishing baits consist of two main groups: natural, which can be anything found in the sea on which fish might normally feed, ranging from a wisp of weed to a whole small crab; and artificial baits which can imitate all the natural baits mentioned above. Strips of fish are also suitable bait.

Coarse fishing baits cover a whole range of items, some of which seem most unlikely. These fish can be caught on the larvae of various kinds of fly (maggots), wasp grubs, seeds of all descriptions including corn-on-the-cob, as well as small fruits such as the elderberry.

Game fishing baits are normally a range of artificial flies, or to be more precise, imitations of real flies (mayflies, caddis, stoneflies . . .) found in or on the water.

Where to fish

There are not many places where there is not some kind of fishable water fairly near. Your local tackle dealer will no doubt be one of your best sources of information. All land adjoining water belongs to someone, that is, apart from that section of the seashore which lies between the high and low tide marks. This means that permission to fish has to be obtained from some person who is responsible for the control of the land. But before one gets permission to go on to land to fish one needs, in the case of game and coarse fishing, to obtain a rod licence. These are issued by the regional Water Authority and can be obtained direct from them or from some tackle dealers who act as agents for the authorities. Fees vary from region to region, but whatever it is a reduction is usually made, subject to certain conditions, for the handicapped angler. Rod licence money is used to maintain and improve fisheries; also many authorities provide special facilities and in some cases special events for those who are handicapped. Rod licences are not required for sea fishing.

Armed with your rod licence one can then set about getting a permit to fish. These can be either on a day basis for a particular water, or a season ticket which might allow you to fish several waters at different places throughout the country. There is also a fishing season – more complications! One can only fish for coarse fish from the 16th June until the 15th March the following year. For game fishing, from October to February no game fish may be taken, but the exact dates vary from region to region. Most Water Authorities produce an annual regional guide which will give you all information on current costs, close seasons, and waters controlled by them. The only thing that these guides might not tell you is whether the fishery is accessible for those who have mobility problems. This problem is slowly being resolved and some Water Authorities will indicate which waters are suitable for the wheelchair user and those who are ambulatory.

Water authorities are, however, only one organisation which provides fishing. There are many organisations which own or control fishing and some produce information about access. These organisations can be statutory bodies such as Local Authorities, Forestry Commission and National Trust, or private bodies such as landowners and angling associations. Just one angling guide is required and some progress has been made. Currently there are three main sources of information on angling facilities that are suitable for the handicapped person: the Regional Water Authorities, the National Anglers' Council and the Country Landowners' Association Charitable Trust.

These by no means cover all the available waters and again the local tackle dealer might be a most useful source of information. If there is still difficulty, do contact the Water Sports Division of the British Sports Association for the Disabled.

How to begin

Angling is unique in many respects, not least of which is the fact that nothing is absolutely certain or positive, other than that if you fall in the water you will get wet! What is right one day may not prove to be so the next. I well remember fishing the River Lea, the river made famous by Isaac Walton's book

The Compleat Angler. It was on a Sunday afternoon. I did not have a lot of time, or bait, and therefore was more than pleased to get over 9 kilos (20 lbs) of good roach, all over 20cm (8 ins) in length (in those days there was a size limit on fish caught), in just over two hours, and even more optimistic about a competition to be held on the same stretch of water the following Tuesday, in which I was taking part. I really thought that I had the match in my hand when I found that I had the same swim on the Tuesday, with the same conditions – bait, water, the weather, everything. I finished in third place with just over 1 kilo (2 lbs) of fish in a six hour match!

You will appreciate, then, that with the different varieties of fish plus the different handicaps that might hinder the angler, there can be no hard and fast methods laid down on how you should fish in order to catch fish. Mind you, that is all to the good. It would be very boring to be able to predict results, and what is more I know from my experience that if I were to say, 'You won't catch fish if you do that,' you can guarantee that someone would do exactly what you suggested they shouldn't and prove you wrong!

All I can do, at this stage, is generalise. Firstly, what are the limitations likely to be imposed on the various disabilities that prospective handicapped anglers might have? Well basically none. I have yet to find a handicapped person who could not fish. Generally it will be up to the individual to decide by trial and error which type or method of angling suits him or her best.

It will not only be the mechanics of the sport that affect a decision. Angling can be all things to all men. Some anglers prefer solitude or just the company of a friend. I well appreciate the pleasure of fishing for tench on an early summer's dawn and watching my float silently lift up through the last wisps of mist lying on the water, knowing that moment is mine alone. Other anglers might be more gregarious and prefer the hustle and bustle of a sea fishing competition from a boat or pier. But whatever you choose, the awesome excitement of deep sea fishing for record shark, or those tense fragments of time as a trout rises to the fly, be assured that of all the outdoor activities angling offers more to a greater number of disabled enthusiasts than any other sport I know.

To reach the best standard that one is capable of requires experience and constant practice, and one never stops learning. You can start fishing at eight and still be finding new twists when you are eighty! To reach your potential as quickly as possible you really need assistance from a qualified instructor of the National Anglers' Council, and to attend angling classes if you can. If this is not possible, do try and get advice from an experienced angler. This is where joining a local angling club can pay dividends, for you can draw on the combined knowledge of the many people who will have fished the waters you will be fishing, and gain socially at the same time.

There is a lot of information available which the individual can obtain for himself, but much of it at first glance may not appear to be directly associated with angling. For example, in the companion book *Out of Doors with Handicapped People* there is in the introduction mention of the weather, wind and water pollution. There is a whole chapter on water and another on the seashore, all of which will help give the prospective angler some background information. The libraries are packed with books on many subjects which all have some bearing on the sport. There are also books dealing directly with many different aspects of the sport itself, from fishing for a particular species such as trout, to fishing specific types of water.

There are three aspects of angling education, each of which is as important as the rest. Firstly, there is the academic side: finding out through books and any other source all that you can absorb on the subjects we have discussed above.

The second aspect is the mechanical one: learning how to operate the various pieces of angling tackle so that the technique becomes automatic – the casting techniques required by different forms of fishing, tying hooks and fixing baits. With both aspects you do not need water and they can be carried out at home. Learning from books you will understand but you can learn the mechanics there as well. Try tying hooks while watching television. Practise casting a small weight into a bucket which is placed further and further away as you improve, and if you have the advantage of sight, try assembling all your angling tackle with your eyes shut.

The third aspect is the practical one, where you go fishing for real, and this also should be a learning experience every time you go out. There is a maxim which says, 'You can't catch a fish with your hook in the air.' This means quite simply that the longer your hook is in the water the more chance you have of catching fish. Yet it is surprising how much time is wasted by lack of practice in, for instance, changing floats or tying a new hook. If you have a chance to watch a top-level angling competition, take a good look at those fishing. It takes a lot of practice to ensure that your bait is in the water, at the right place, for as long as possible in the time that is available!

Who can fish?
Whatever your handicap, you should never state what you cannot do, only emphasise what you can do. I personally am not concerned with the handicapped angler, but rather with the angler who has a handicap.

If you have reasonable use of both arms and hands, whether or not you are in a wheelchair, this means that you can compete on equal terms with other anglers, provided of course that access is no problem. I know many paraplegics and single and double leg amputees who are members of angling clubs and in fact represent those clubs in competitions. If you only have use of one arm then there can be some problems with using a rod and reel, although I know of single arm flyfishers who regularly fish with a fly, an occupation which is normally associated with the use of both arms. This is achieved, after practice, by the use of a harness which is strapped to the body and holds the rod. There are lots of examples: the use of hook holders and the like. If you have an artificial arm then again you are on a par with those with use of both. There are lots of attachments that are of help; I know of two single arm fishermen who are qualified angling instructors. Fishing with the pole is ideal if you are going coarse fishing and you can, in fact, dap a fly on the water for trout if this is allowed in your area.

Visually handicapped anglers usually find that ledgering suits them best. In this normal ledgering tackle is used, the ledger cast out, the rod placed on rod rests and the line tightened up. Bites can then be felt by just touching the line. There are audible bite indicators on the market for those who prefer them. The use of lures and spinners, as well as the fly, can also be useful methods of catching fish, as all these rely to some extent on touch. In a recent trout fishing match a totally blind angler was judged to be the best of the day; he located rising fish by the sound they made and caught them on a fly.

The hearing impaired have no problems, providing the balance is not affected. The only snag that I have come across, and it's not serious, is in taking part in open competitions when the start and end of the match is normally indicated by a whistle being blown – an easily solved problem.

Mentally handicapped anglers differ only in the degree of handicap. Simple pole fishing for coarse fishing or line fishing at the seaside are quite possibly the best methods for the majority, but there are individuals who very easily master the techniques of spinning and casting. The only point to be made is that adequate supervision must be maintained, for all those who participate in angling, handicapped or not, should realise that it is a risk sport and care should always be taken.

Epilepsy is no problem, but it is strongly recommended that anyone who might be subject to an attack should fish with some other person who is aware of the problem and can render assistance should it be required.

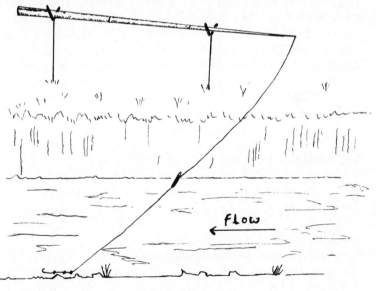

'Laying on'

Those who have difficulty in holding or gripping will also find that they get results by fishing with a pole which should be as long as the individual can manage, and using a method known as 'laying on'. This method can only be employed for coarse fishing but in any type of water. It is a combination of float and ledger fishing: the hook and float are cast out and the rod placed on rod rests; the float will come to rest downstream of the pole tip. However, although conventional float tackle is used, the line from the float to the hook is 30 or 60cm (1 or 2ft) longer than the depth of water. With very little practice this can become a most effective way of fishing. The same method can be used by those who have poor co-ordination or those who are unable to lift even the lightest type of rod for short periods of time. With anyone who has problems with grip, or with holding or lifting, it has been found that, if the angler sits at right angles to the water and places the rod or pole also at right angles, then the base of the rod or pole – the butt end – presents itself in a better manner. The use of thermal plastic or any other material on the butt end, shaped to the individual's needs, is always an advantage.

The severely handicapped require equipment which often is not readily available. It usually has to be made to individual specific requirements and as a result can be expensive. It is a fact, however, that anyone who can manipulate an electric driven wheelchair can fish to some extent, and I know of a quadriplegic who uses a possum device attached to electronic gearing: sipping in starts the reel revolving while a puff stops it. For these more severely handicapped anglers the tasks of baiting up, casting and landing fish caught do have to be carried out by an assistant and one who preferably has some knowledge of the sport.

The approach of anyone who contemplates taking up the sport should always be positive. One should not say, 'Can I fish?' but 'How will I fish?'

Interests associated with angling
It has been said before that there's more to angling than catching fish. All clubs have officials and committees that manage and look after the affairs of the club, but angling clubs do have a much wider range of responsibility than the average

sports club. Sea fish and game fish are part of any country's food resources and to a lesser degree so are some species of coarse fish. This means that there are all kinds of rules and regulations governing the catching of fish, the methods employed, the size of fish that are allowed to be retained, notification of diseases, control of pollution. The Ministry of Agriculture and Fisheries has regulations, as do the Water Authorities, the Common Market, Local Authorities and so on. Although it might seem to be rather involved, it can be very interesting work. The honorary club secretary and the treasurer are invaluable in dealing with such items as negotiating fishing leases, restocking with fish, buying fishing craft, fighting rate demands, getting grant aid for development – all of which are part and parcel of the angling scene.

The point that I am trying to make is that you do not have to be an angler to get involved in the sport. Other interests that you might have could prove to be an asset. An interest in photography and writing could fit you for the post of Press and Public Relations Officer. In fact there are very few interests outside angling that cannot be related to the sport.

Another aspect of angling that is of interest to many is the construction of some of the many items of angling equipment one uses. Fly tying for game fishing is a prime example, but there is also the manufacturing of floats, rods, rod rests, tackle boxes, lures and spinners. If one becomes proficient in the production of any of these items one can readily establish a small home business.

Practical fishing costs
The cost of angling is increasing – in some areas rapidly. I am often asked the question, 'What will it cost me?' and I find it hard to reply. Prices for a rod and reel can vary as much as the difference in price between a Mini and a Rolls Royce. All I can say is that, whatever your cash limits, you will be able to afford some angling equipment sufficient to allow you to undertake the type and method of fishing to suit you.

Other variations which affect the cost are transport and licences; how often you might go fishing and how far that fishing is from where you live. But there are ways and means by which you can help to reduce those items which are essential.

Rod licences from Water Authorities are often reduced in cost for the handicapped person, so make enquiries. Fishing tickets are far cheaper if you belong to a local club that has its own water rather than purchasing day tickets. Some angling associations offer good value for money on their season tickets, but this needs some consideration to discover which type of fishing ticket is best for you. How often shall I be able to go fishing? How far away is the water? These are just two questions that you need to consider. If you can only fish a couple or so times a year, then it's a day ticket for you. If you can fish every day of every week then it's a club season ticket. Some clubs have only one water, some have several, some clubs are affiliated to angling associations which might have a great many waters, and then you get back to transport.

The more times you go out the more it costs. Joining a club can help with transport costs for they can be shared, bearing in mind that if it's a coarse fishing club, two anglers might be the limit for the average car if you have to take a wheelchair. Some clubs have their own coach transport, others hire coaches for special trips. But these are only viable where there are sufficient regular members consistently to fill the coach. Some of the more enlightened Local Authorities provide transport for the handicapped, or if you have a large number of juniors it might be worth while affiliating to the local Youth and Community Service, or its equivalent.

Hooks can be purchased tied or untied, in small amounts or large. Buying them tied is the most expensive, buying them untied in boxes of 100 is the cheapest. The only problem is that you need hooks of different sizes and perhaps types, which could mean that you might finish up with a thousand hooks or so. Not much saving in the short term in that! But if you have a group who all want hooks you can combine your needs. Local clubs, buying in bulk from a local tackle dealer, also attract a discount.

Line in bulk purchase makes this item cheaper, too. Most anglers buy 100 or 200 metres at a time. The same line can be bought in 1,000 metres or even more in some cases. There are instances where a different weight of line might be required for a particular type of fishing. To cater for this, most reels have two spools and spare ones can be purchased. This is fine, but to

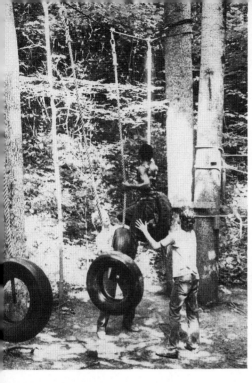

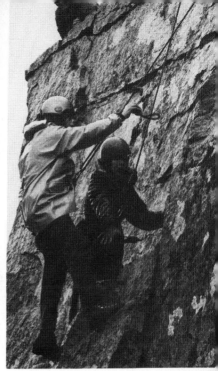

Levels of adventure

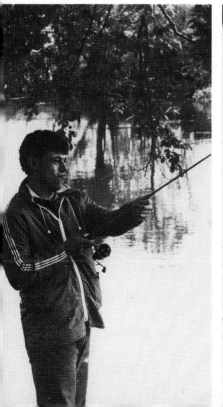

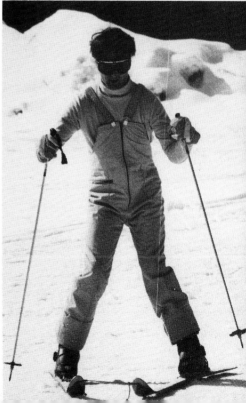

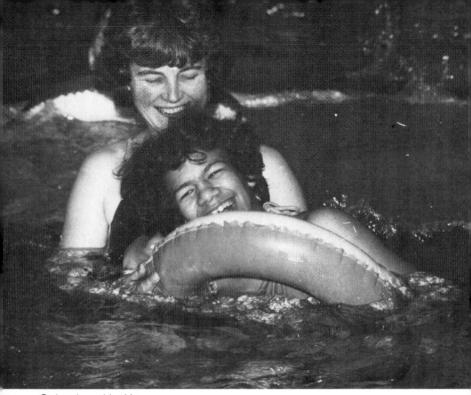

Swimming with aids

Splashing about

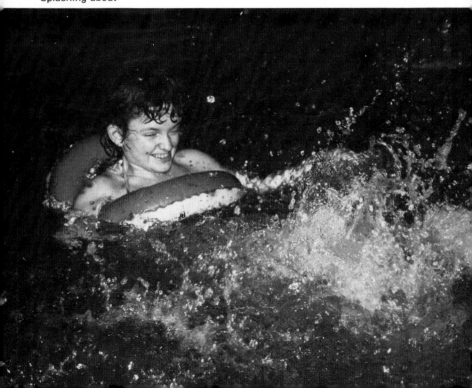

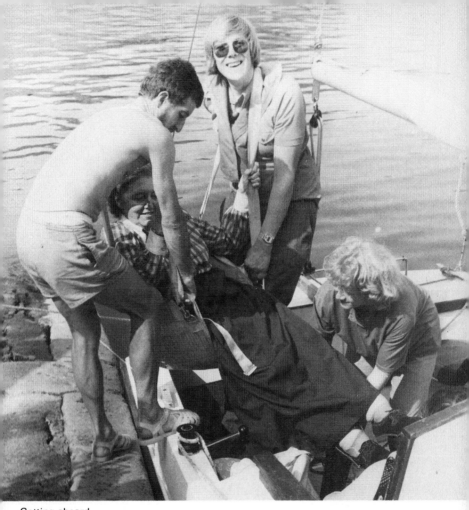

Getting aboard

Dinghy sailing

Handling the tiller

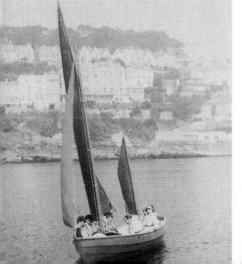

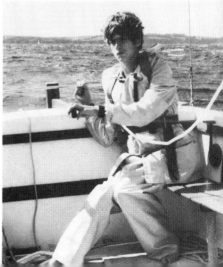

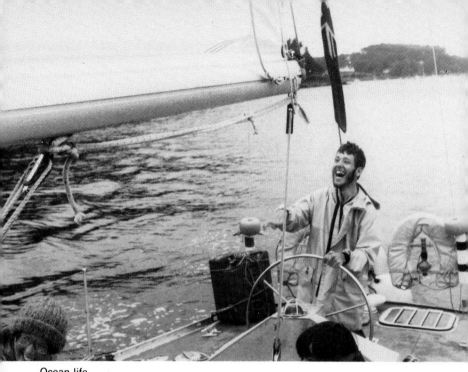

Ocean life

Cruising holiday

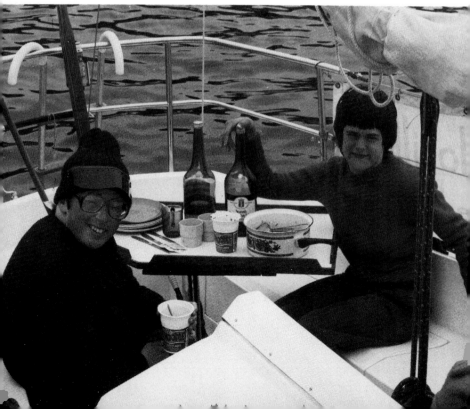

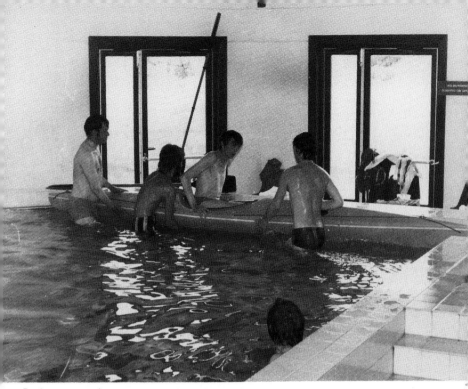

Pool canoe session

Beach launch

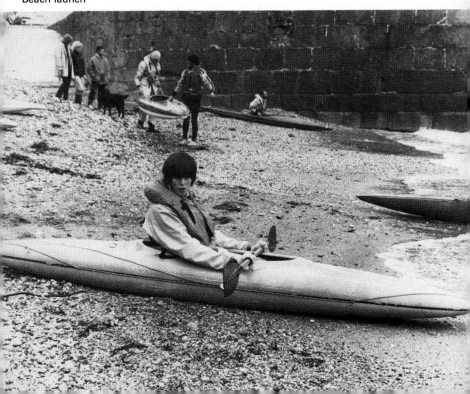

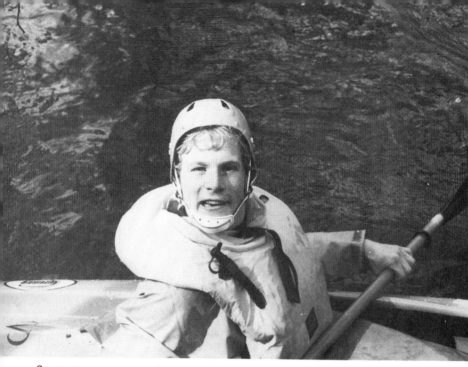

Canoe gear

Introducing the caranoe

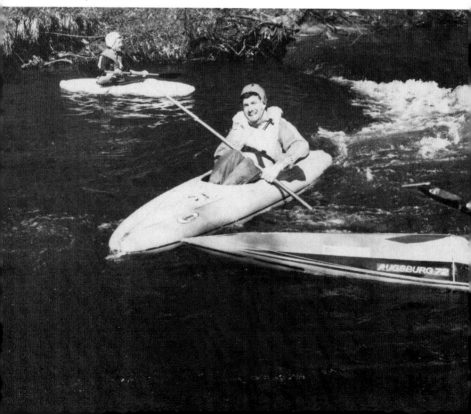

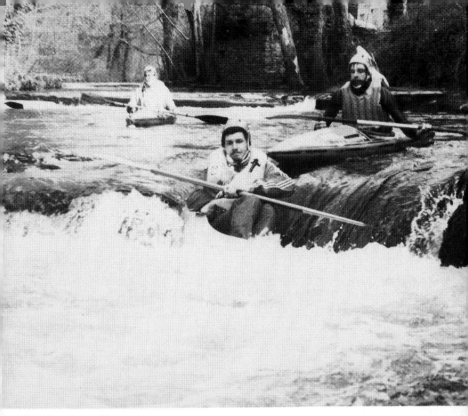

Running the rapids

Canadian canoe adventure

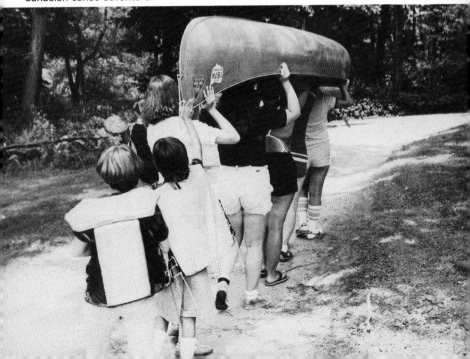

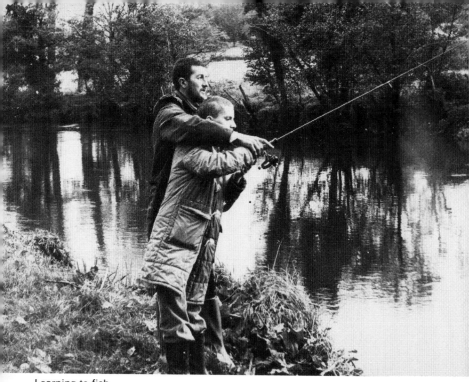

Learning to fish

River solitude

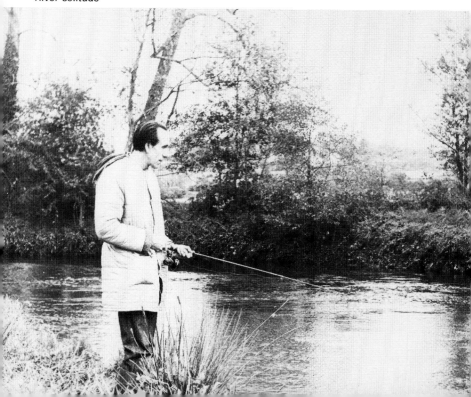

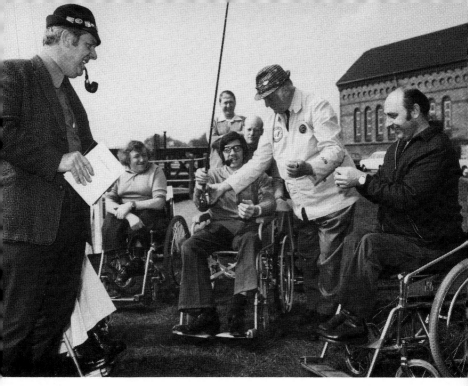

Instruction in game fishing

Beginning indoors

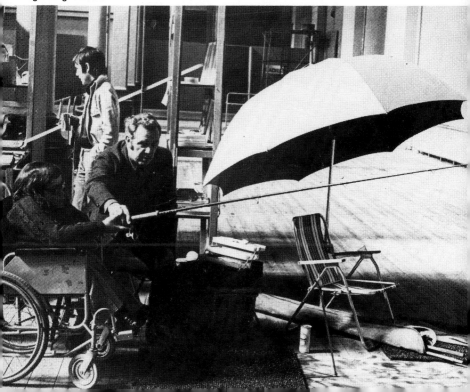

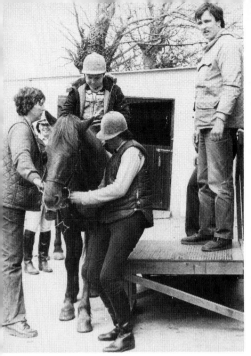

Help in mounting

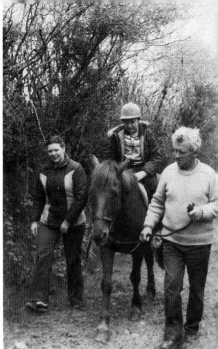

A country ride

A riding holiday

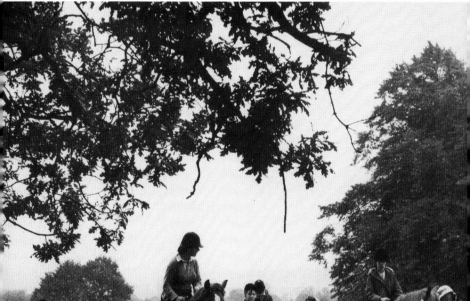

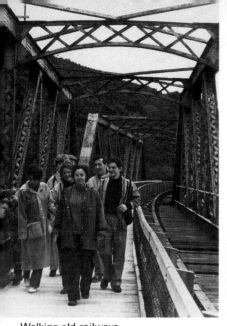

Walking old railways

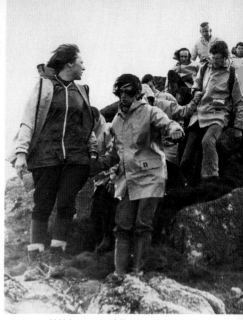

Wild country hikes

On top of the world

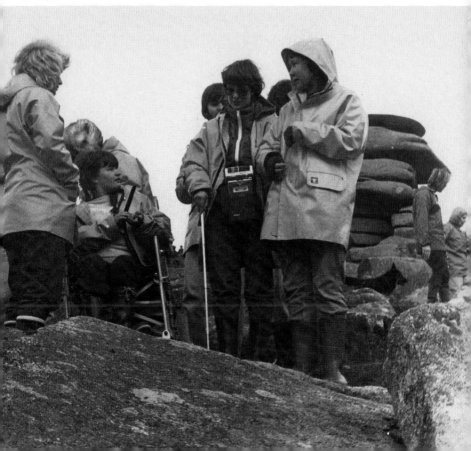

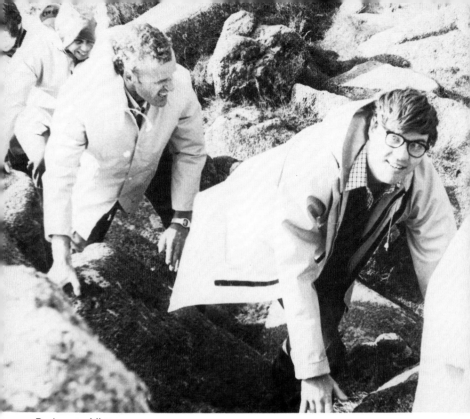

Rock scrambling

Rough country for sticks

The end of the course

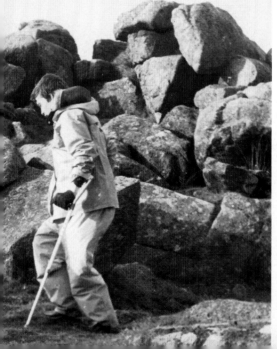

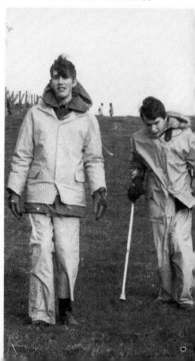

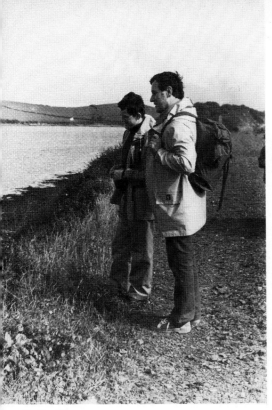

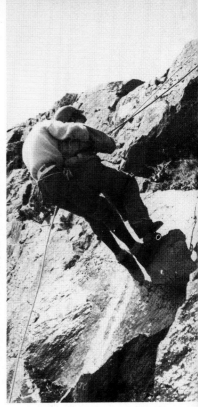

Backpacking

Abseiling

Alpine expedition

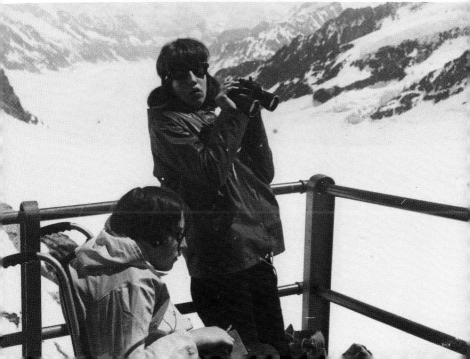

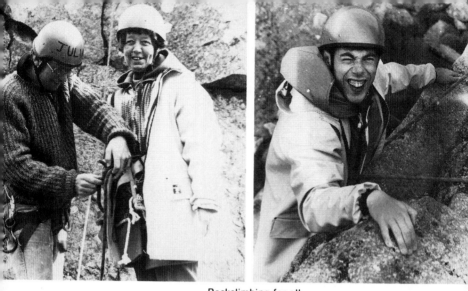

Rockclimbing for all

Determination

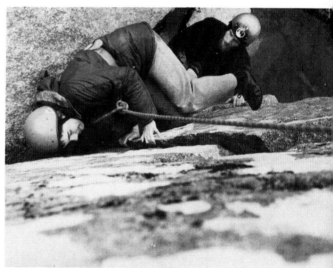

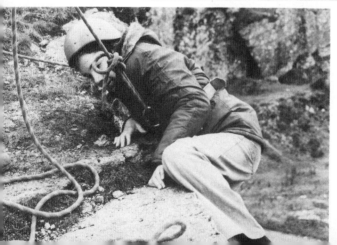

Reaching the top

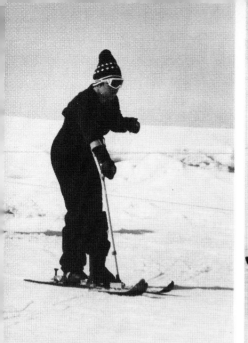

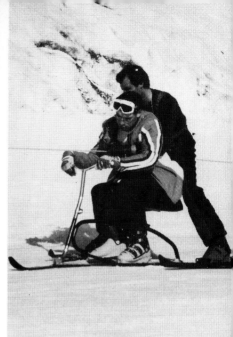

Ski with an outrigger

Ski bobbing

Help balance with the pole

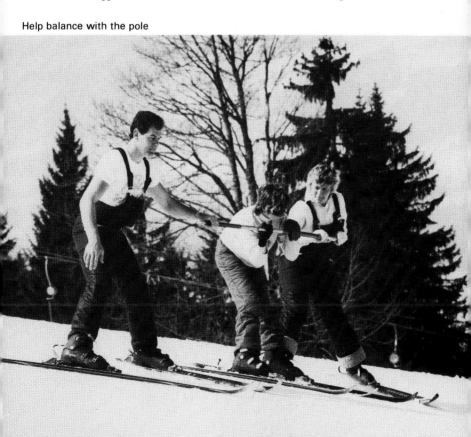

Winter fun on
American camps

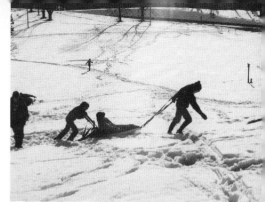

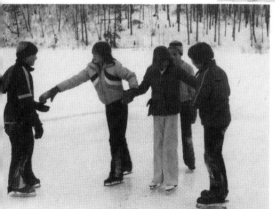

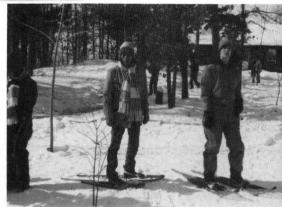

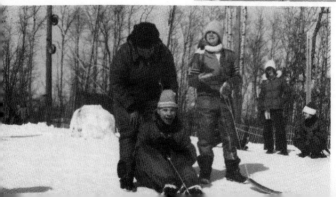

fill all the reels with all the types of line you might wish to use could prove costly. Depending on the type of fishing you intend to do, have a line which is most likely to be used on one of the spools – for the sake of example, let's presume it is 1 kilo (2 lbs). On the other reel we could have 2.25 kilo (5 lb) line. By tying hooks on line, that are of other breaking strains below the 2.25 kilo spool we can have a range of lines from as low as 227g (½ lb) up to 2.25 kilos. I personally have two freshwater reels, each with two spools, and I can fish right up to 5.50 kilo (12 lb) breaking strain or down 454g (1 lb) at a time to 454g line. It's a lot cheaper that way.

Floats come in all shapes and sizes and can be costly. With patience, however, many of them can be made for a few pence. In fact, if you can obtain various sizes of feathers, they need not cost you anything. Old corks from medicine bottles and the like can be shaped and a hole drilled through them to hold your quills, to give you heavier floats. If you feel that you require a more sophisticated float for a particular type of water, then pieces of cane and balsa can usually provide the material. Not everyone feels that they are up to the mark when it comes to making a good quality item but we solved this in one of my clubs by a group getting together and deciding which floats would suit each member and then each person doing just one job. One would measure and cut the pieces, another would rub them roughly into shape, and so on with each person doing what they were capable of; it worked well and saved a lot of money!

Most rods and poles are made in glass fibre which if looked after will last almost a lifetime. Carbon fibre is also used and although it's much lighter and stronger it is also much more expensive. One way of keeping costs down, and this is the same for reels, is for the club to decide what make or type it wants and then buy them in bulk. Another way of even further reducing the costs of rods and poles is to purchase the blanks that make up the body of the rod, plus the rings and reel fittings, and then make up the rods at home or at the club.

These are just a few suggestions. There are many other ways in which the angler with a little imagination can keep costs down to a reasonable level. The biggest problem is that everything mentioned above presumes that one is going to take up the sport in earnest; but how to provide equipment for possible new members who as yet are not sure that this is the sport for them? Most angling tackle is a personal thing and anglers do not like to lend rods, reels and tackle. One of my junior clubs solved this particular problem by investing in the basic requirements and hiring to the newcomer at a very low fee. If the individual decided he wanted to take up the sport he would buy the equipment he had been using at the cost to the club, less half of the amount he had paid in hiring fees. Any scheme on these lines can soon be established.

You may have noticed that in itemising the basic gear I left out the landing net. This was not an oversight. If you are in a club situation it's almost certain that there will be others with landing nets close at hand when you might need one. The keepnet was included for the simple reason that most groups compete against each other and in these circumstances the keep net is essential. There is not a lot that one can do about making the actual nets used. They have to be of knotless netting, and being made from nylon they do not rot. The handles and rod rests, however, are a different matter. The connecting points on this type of equipment are screw fittings and they all have the same diameter. I have seen the screw fitting put onto all kinds of things to make a rod rest or bank stick for the keep net. Old rods that have been broken and can no longer be used as such do make good landing net handles, provided that the length you have is strong enough.

If you happen to need a particular piece of equipment that is either too expensive to buy or simply not available, why not try your local school? If they have metal and wood working shops you will quite often find that the teacher in charge might be only too happy to give some of his pupils the chance to make something out of the normal run.

So the costs need not deter you from trying your luck at angling and, who knows, you may well find you enjoy it so much that you have an interest for life. With rod in hand beside the water's edge, the sight of a fish in the river before you, there can be few more peaceful and yet exciting ways in which to spend the day.

5   In the saddle

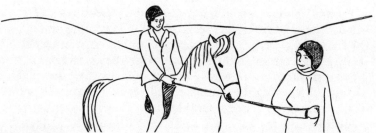

Introduction

The horse and pony offer something unique to the physically handicapped person, a set of real legs that can take him further and faster than he can go on his own, and that can become almost an extension of himself. Here is a mobility that depends neither on mechanical contrivances nor on human pushing power. While at first all his energies may be concentrated on adapting to the movement pattern, on staying upright on this large creature so far from the ground, with proper teaching and help, before very long he can be having the greater satisfaction of learning to control it himself, of becoming a rider instead of a passenger.

Consider for a moment the reasons why riding has such charms for the able-bodied. There is the exhilaration of covering the ground on something large and strong that responds to commands and will do as one asks, but has a will and character of its own. All muscles are exercised and the actual exercise gives a feeling of well being. There is the satisfaction of developing the skill necessary, at first just to keep control, later to jump fences, to ask bigger questions of the horse and to perform more complicated movements more elegantly. This often leads to a desire to compete against others, to test one's skill and ability. For some, lacking the competitive urge, to have achieved a satisfactory working partnership with the horse is enough and they are content to enjoy seeing the countryside from an equine back and to have found a delightful means of locomotion. Almost all find that the horse is a great friend maker, that shared experience and 'horsey talk' is fun. Last, but certainly not least, there is the pleasure to be found in the company of the horse himself, an animal that has so much to give and that has served man generously down the centuries.

For the handicapped rider the potential pleasures are just the same, but magnified. His everyday mobility is more limited, so the freedom given is more of a privilege. His chances of taking stimulating exercise in the fresh air, which he greatly needs, are more restricted, and this way he can take it sitting down. The process of learning the necessary skills may be a very slow one if his handicap is considerable, but there is even greater challenge; and when this is accepted and the right help given, he can learn to use what ability he has, and may well with the special incentive find he can achieve far more than he expected. Competitions graded to his ability can be open to him, and if these do not appeal, the new access he has to places where wheelchairs and buses will not go opens up a whole new world. He finds friends, not just among those who share the lessons, but with the able-bodied who help him, and to whom he can express views born of his experience, as well as listen to theirs. Probably having had little chance of intimate contact with animals, he makes the delightful discovery that, properly handled, a horse can become a friend as well as a conveyance. For many mentally handicapped children and adults, as well as for those physically handicapped who are withdrawn and cut off from other people by communication difficulties, to form a relationship with a living creature that demands respect but responds to affection and understanding is of very special value, and can draw out and make the forming of relationships with other humans less difficult.

Having said this, we must be careful not to make it sound too idyllic, too easy, and to give the impression (as is sometimes given) that all that needs to be done to achieve spectacular results is to pick an amiable looking pony, seat the disabled person on its back, attach an attendant, and wait for the miracle.

The rider who is struggling to stay upright in an uncomfortable saddle several sizes too small for him, towed along by someone whose mind is on other matters and whose one idea is to get round the field three times and then change her passenger, to whom he cannot communicate his desire to stop and relieve the pinching of his knees by the stirrup irons through thin trousers, is certainly not developing confidence or having much pleasure. The enthusiastic lady who comes from behind with shouts of encouragement and who in her anxiety to prevent him slipping off to the right, with a hefty heave nearly sends him off to the left, increases rather than decreases his anxiety. It is the last straw when the pony, innocently enough, puts its head down to snatch at a tempting bit of grass and the front end suddenly seems to disappear, wrenching the reins out of his hands. He may, once safely on the ground again, derive some satisfaction from having been through such an unfamiliar experience and survived the ordeal, but he has certainly not had a happy introduction to the joys of horsemanship or developed any sense of being master of his fate.

There is no question about it, if riding is to give pleasure, do good, and be conducted safely a great deal of expertise, attention to detail, and understanding of the disabled person's problems is required. This does not mean that the lesson should be an over-serious, intense affair. It should above all give fun and satisfaction in which the pupils and teachers share. The fun will be immeasurably the greater if teaching techniques are sound and everyone feels safe and comfortable. The teaching of riding to anyone with special difficulties, whether resulting from physical or mental handicap, must therefore be undertaken by those who have sufficient knowledge of both riding and handicap, though these may not necessarily be those who will be the most successful at polishing up the able-bodied 'star turn' riders for high powered competition.

The horse and pony
There is clearly one big difference between the teaching of riding and the teaching of other outdoor activities: the extra personality of the pony is introduced into the proceedings. (The word 'pony' from now on should be taken as covering horse or pony, as in fact far more ponies than horses are useful for the handicapped rider.) He is a living creature with his own likes and dislikes, a capacity for being hurt, frightened, upset and awkward, and his good or bad behaviour affects the teaching situation all the time. Although all ponies have some characteristics in common, each one is an individual with his

own idiosyncracies and needs to be respected as such and handled correctly if he is to serve as a co-operative partner. Sound 'horse sense' on the part of those who handle him is the best safeguard against avoiding accidents and agitations.

By no means all ponies are suitable for beginners, let alone for handicapped people. Some are too excitable, some too nervous, some too obstinate, and some lack the necessary training. The very sluggish, however safe, may give so little response to the rider's requests that scant progress can be made on them, although they may be adequate for first lessons. A good, kind, calm temperament is the first essential, and sufficient training for the job the second. Those used must stand still to be mounted, lead quietly and willingly, be good tempered with others, and not have bad habits of biting or kicking. Young ponies under five years old, however promising, should not be used as they lack the reliability that only comes with maturity, but the very ancient and decrepit make depressing and even unsafe mounts. The lethargy that results from under-feeding and lack of condition must not be mistaken for the true quietness we are looking for. Lame and sick animals must not be used, and surely no handicapped rider would knowingly want his pleasure to be taken at the price of causing distress or pain.

The pony must be of a suitable size for the rider. Short human legs stretched across huge fat equine backs, or long legs reaching almost to the ground from a small pony, make the rider's difficulties greater. Heavy riders, extra-heavy because they sit mounted on a saddle, on ponies not up to their weight, can cause strain and sore backs. Most riders are best suited by the compact, 'cobby' type of pony which provides a more solid base to sit on and has less rapid movements than those of more quality type. But some riders with adductor spasm are more comfortable on narrow ponies; some ponies are upset by certain riders but will go kindly for others – reactions must be watched and changes made if necessary. The big horse makes it difficult for dismounted helpers to reach up to assist the rider when required; his stride tends to be too long for comfort, and sheer distance from the ground makes for anxiety. Most adults can be satisfactorily mounted on the larger of the native pony breeds and on sturdy cobs not exceeding 15 hands. It may prove impossible to mount the exceptionally outsize rider, who may have an incentive to lose weight if he wants to take up riding.

The choice of pony is therefore a very important matter and must be made by those with sound horse knowledge, as well as experience of the problems created by disability. It is better to provide worthwhile riding for a few than to attempt to press into action those animals that are fundamentally unsuitable, in the absence of sufficient acceptable ones. It is only the contented healthy pony who serves the disabled rider well.

Saddlery and equipment

On grounds of safety, and to ensure comfort of both riders and ponies, all saddlery must be kept in good condition and must be fitted correctly. Any old saddle will emphatically not do; the discomfort caused by a really bad saddle or one that is too small for a bulky rider has to be experienced to be believed. Here again the experienced eye and great care in saddling up are necessary. But responsible riders, even if disabled, can and should learn to understand the essentials and to check up many points themselves.

It is very important that stirrup irons be of the correct size. Nothing is more dangerous than irons too small so that feet can become wedged in them, and those that are far too large are almost as bad, as feet can slip right through and ankles become caught. Peacock open-sided safety irons with thick rubber bands, although expensive, are very desirable and especially so when riders have reached the stage of being off the leading rein and are out in the open, when inevitably the odd fall becomes more likely.

A pony must always be lead by a leading rein attached to a well fitted head collar, never by the reins. Certain strong mounts may need to be lead from the bit, but this should be by means of a divided leading rein that snaps on to both rings, never by fastening the rein to one ring and passing it through the other. Soft rope leading reins and adjustable head collars are not expensive and, in cases where the pony owners cannot provide them, should be taken along by those organising the riding.

Other simple items of equipment that should be available are handles and/or neck straps that can be used by the rider in emergency and to give security. There are various designs. These will discourage the rider from hanging on to the pony's mouth by the reins. Another generally useful item is the grass rein which prevents a pony getting his head down to eat grass and which can consist simply of string passed from bit rings to saddle 'D's' via the corner of the browband. And mention should be made here of the popular 'safety belt', an adjustable webbing belt with handle on the back which goes round the rider's waist and which the dismounted helper can hold when necessary. This is better called an 'emergency belt'. It can indeed be useful in moments of crisis and can give confidence to anxious riders and helpers in the early stages, but it was never designed, as it is often used, for 'strap hanging'. Improperly used, by being grasped all the time, it can unbalance a rider and restrict rather than encourage progress.

There are a number of other items of special equipment that help in individual cases, some of which have been contrived after much experimenting, but equipment of this kind should only be resorted to when it provides the only answer, and the simpler it is the better. In no case should anything be used which in any way ties the rider to the horse, and complicated gadgetry which makes the rider feel different from other people is to be avoided.

Sheepskin saddle covers, securely fastened, can be a great comfort to those riders liable to pressure sores. Soft felt pads instead of leather saddles suit some small riders. Australian stock saddles, and certain types of Western saddles, help a number of riders, especially when riding for longer periods than usual, as on holiday, but they are not often available in this country.

Clothes
Equipping the rider is easier. Expensive riding clothes are not necessary, although protective head wear and suitable shoes are essentials. For the rest, although jodpurs may give the wearer much satisfaction, they often prove difficult for the physically handicapped to get on and off, and thick jeans or suitably cut slacks that do not ride up are quite adequate, together with jerseys and/or windcheaters. Track suits are

often found comfortable. Avoid anything that flaps or clutters up the rider, and remember that some ponies dislike the crackle of certain types of waterproof material. Feet and hands often get cold, so warm socks and non-slip gloves should not be forgotten in cold weather.

The necessity for protecting the head from possible injury is now universally accepted, although some able-bodied riders still foolishly choose to ignore this. There has been much discussion, and much experimental work is going on, regarding the design and structure of riding caps and the best way to keep them on the head in case of a fall, but the carefully fitted velvet covered cap with flexible peaks, with its conventional appearance, is regarded as satisfactory for everyday riding provided that it does stay on. Those with exceptionally large heads may need specially made helmets. A good fit is the first essential; a hat that shifts when the rider shakes his head is useless. There are various types of chin straps, but a wide elastic band under the chin is generally more comfortable. Old hats are often given by kindly people for use by disabled riders but these should be examined carefully to make sure that they have not suffered from damage in the past – squashy ones are useless. Where hats have to be worn by a variety of riders, fit can be improved by inserting strips of foam rubber in the lining, but where riders have moved on past the beginner stage, and so are indulging in greater activity, it is ideal if each can have his own cap that fits him exactly.

Although heads may be protected, bad footwear all too often passes unnoticed. Shoes must be flat heeled, strong and simple with reasonably smooth soles. High heeled ones, those with buckles or trimmings that may catch in stirrup irons, open sandals, plimsolls, and rubber boots with rough corrugated soles are all dangerous, as they may get caught up.

Where to ride
An enclosed flat space, protected from traffic noise, other horses and other distractions and as far as possible from wind (which can have a dramatic effect on ponies) is essential for lessons. The surface must be suitable, ie. not concrete, rutty, or a sea of mud, and the use of an all-weather surfaced manege, or better still, a covered school clearly makes life much easier. The

covered school can not only be used in all weather but its walls give a sense of security and make for concentration; in it riders can usually be allowed off the leading rein sooner, and progress be achieved more quickly.

Perfect facilities, however, are not always available; an imaginative instructor can do wonders in less than ideal conditions, but the open space of a common or the grass verge of a road are not the place for lessons. At a later stage there will be a need to get out and about and access to short rides on tracks and through woodland is then very desirable. Riding on any roads presents hazards and even when one road has to be crossed or ridden along for short distances good safety precautions must be taken, with helpers sent ahead or to the rear to slow traffic down if necessary. In due course, however, riders who are going to be able to get out and around must learn road sense, as it affects riding like everyone else, and they should be taught to express thanks to motorists who show consideration.

Mounting

To sit in a wheelchair and view an apparently gigantic animal looming above can produce a certain sense of despair – not so much if one is a small child whom willing arms will lift on board, but certainly if one weighs thirteen stone and has little physical power to help oneself. The business of mounting can also cause agitation, and back strain on the part of the helpers, and with wheelchairs and crutches getting in everyone's way can indeed be an anxious business. But to get the riders 'on board' is indeed the first essential. It must be tackled methodically and with thought behind it, if the ride is to start off happily.

The first essential is that the ponies should have been taught to stand quite still beside, and to come up close to, mounting blocks or ramps without viewing these with suspicion – an aspect of training all too often neglected. There is nothing more disconcerting to a handicapped person than to be hauled or lifted onto a heaving mass of horse that is being unwillingly anchored by several people imploring it to 'whoa!' One person should hold the pony firmly but in a relaxed way, standing in front of him, while others attend to the needs of the rider. There are various lifting methods which are better demonstrated than described, and which an experienced instructor or physiotherapist can teach. Some riders will depend entirely on being lifted, but whenever possible each should be encouraged to help himself as far as he can, and with encouragement can do more than is expected. Adults should be mounted with as much dignity as possible, and may have definite views about the form of help they want; no one likes being treated as a sack of coal with the 'one, two, three heave' approach.

How to mount all sizes and types of rider without fuss and with the minimum effort for everyone requires learning. Never forget that it can take a long time to get everybody up and comfortably settled and relaxed, with stirrups correctly adjusted, before the lesson is ready to begin.

From beginnings to achievements
In the early stages each rider is likely to need a helper walking on either side of him, as well as someone to lead the pony. Thus riding for the disabled is heavily dependent on a considerable amount of man/woman power, the supply of which is often the limiting factor. It is a very rewarding field of service, although quite taxing physically, and as suitable for older teenagers as for the pony-loving mothers who so often oblige. Of whatever age, helpers must learn the right methods, be prepared to come regularly so that riders get to know and trust them, and do as the instructor or physiotherapist requests. Careless, inattentive helpers can create dangers, and bored ones reduce the value of the riding. The aim is, however, to reduce gradually the riders' reliance on helpers as far as possible, developing the confidence, balance and suppleness which will enable them to learn to 'ride properly' – in some cases this may be a very slow process with the breakthrough coming after weeks or months of patiently plodding on. Independent riding can be much more easily achieved where circumstances are favourable and ponies well trained and responsive.

A well conducted lesson should include demonstration, much activity, carefully chosen exercises, games and some gentle stretching of mind and body combined with enjoyment. Clearly there should be a different approach to a small heavily handicapped cerebral palsy child, a robust but severely retarded adolescent, a fit young adult facing up to life without a limb after an accident, and a middle aged person who has had a stroke. It will be a great advantage to have the help occasionally, if not always, of a physiotherapist who can assess the physical problems and advise on the particular methods and exercises that can help each individual, as well as giving the instructor confidence.

One of the most common questions asked is, 'How much risk is involved?' The first safeguard is to have medical permission for each rider. A few conditions may contra-indicate riding, and others may require special care. All safety precautions must be carried out and constant watch kept for signs of fatigue and strain. But as with any active sport a small element of risk remains, and if it is reasonably small, must be accepted. Once he has advanced to being free from dismounted helpers no one can guarantee that a rider will never fall off. If the moment comes when he feels he wants to attempt the canter and the instructor is satisfied that he is ready for it the plunge must be taken, and both rider and instructor must take the risk, otherwise no going forward is possible. Foolish accidents caused by mismanagement, unsafe equipment and lack of foresight can always be prevented.

Without enlarging on the principles of horsemanship, the basic riding skills, reduced to the simplest terms, consist of learning to stay on, start, steer and stop, keeping comfortable and not causing the pony discomfort. The burden of disability born by some people is such that however carefully they are taught they cannot get very far in developing these skills, and will always have to rely heavily on dismounted helpers. They can nevertheless develop self esteem and confidence, have the pleasure of looking down from a pony's back rather than up from a wheelchair, enjoy for a short time their new-found mobility and the games it enables them to play with others, and learn much, even though it is not strictly all about riding. Even when riding does not lead far or last long, their limited experience will have been enriched, and there need be no feeling of failure that they do not actually make riding progress.

Many more can go much further and, with the right help, develop abilities that can compensate for disabilities, finding that in the absence of tension through trying too hard they will discover ways of pressing many of the 'right buttons'. They will be able to control ponies and indulge in considerable riding activity, even though they may always need a sheltered environment and skilled help. And a few will emerge who will break through the barriers and surprise themselves and everyone else by reaching the stage where they can hold their own with the able-bodied, their handicaps left behind while they are in the saddle. Who can measure achievement?

Holidays

Few handicapped riders will get more than one regular riding session each week. The great joy of a riding holiday is that at last they have continuity, riding each day for perhaps a whole week, with the chance to get to know the ponies much better and to develop confidence from day to day. If they can be involved with the care of the ponies so much the better. But even though the riding is the central feature round which the programme is built, the theme should be one of discovery, of exploring fresh places to find new interests. The holiday is a wonderful chance to open eyes and ears and to widen horizons.

The Riding for the Disabled Association has been organising holidays for its riders of all ages for ten years, both at national and local level. Although a few of these take the form of short courses for the more ambitious who want to concentrate on improvement, the majority are more in the nature of modified trekking holidays where formal instruction is left behind and the emphasis is on fun and exploration of a new countryside. Clearly safety precautions cannot be left behind and standards must not be lowered, but although help and advice will still be needed, especially in new circumstances, leaders and participants are all on holiday together and the learning comes from experiencing new situations and facing different challenges from those in the familiar riding school at home. Many people return not only with riding confidence much boosted but having also had a glimpse of a much wider world and all that it offers. From a pony's back one has a good chance to see birds, beasts and trees and so much more, and perhaps to wonder at them for the first time.

Several centres for the disabled now also offer holidays

which include riding, either as a main or subsidiary feature. Commercial Trekking Centres are increasingly prepared to cater for the needs of handicapped parties, though not usually during the peak season. It is vital, however, to make certain on a preliminary visit that facilities are suitable, the ponies of the right type, that the welcome will be genuine and special needs understood.

Where riders are mounted for the first time on unfamiliar ponies there may be some increased anxiety and tension. Very careful fitting of riders to mounts is essential, and once a partnership is established it should, if possible, be maintained for the whole holiday. The wide open spaces can also produce unexpected anxiety, so do not expect too much on the first day. In those cases where the ponies themselves are brought from home to a strange place, remember that they too can react unexpectedly – the one who is perfect in an enclosed school may prove too free and enthusiastic when faced with open moorland. Seasoned trekking ponies who carry novices all summer are usually well disciplined and used to the job of proceeding in single file, even though they may not give the lightest or most responsive of rides.

The most common problem encountered by the rider on a trekking holiday is that of becoming overtired and sore. Bruised and broken skin on legs and seats can end in sheer misery, and with some disabilities serious problems can result. To ride all day including going up and down hill is a very different matter from spending an hour in a school. Only the toughest riders can cope with this – for most a couple of hours will be sufficient, and great care must be taken that no one is overtaxed – comfortably stretched, yes, but certainly not exhausted. Riders should not be accepted unless they have been riding regularly in recent weeks, and allowance must be made for the strains imposed by very hot or very wet weather.

In planning the programme the organiser must have clearly in mind the type of rider for whom he is catering: those who are proficient enough to ride off a leading rein, with mounted leaders and helpers, those who can lead from other horses, or those who must have helpers on foot. Clearly the distances that can be covered when the dismounted helpers are needed will be much less than where everyone is mounted, and those on foot must face up to the fact that plodding up hill and down dale is harder going than round school or paddock. Helpers are not superhuman, and driving them to the point of exhaustion does not help the smooth running of a holiday. Where lead horses are used these also must be quiet and used to leading and those riding them competent enough to deal with emergencies.

The organiser must have full details in advance of the experience, fitness and problems of each rider and must be firm in refusing to take anyone who is unlikely to be able to cope. One overfaced rider can wreck a holiday if all the plans have to be changed to suit his needs, and one bored and frustrated rider who feels he is being held back can be a disappointed, awkward customer to deal with. Inevitably there will be some differences in staying power and skills, however; everyone must be prepared for some give and take.

The severely handicapped rider who needs a lot of help must not be forgotten, but he will need the lesser adventure, and the round of a few fields and woodland paths will suit him better than the great spaces of the Welsh mountains. Even on the most modest holiday each ride can be made into something of an expedition and each small hill become an Everest! A picnic lunch can be as much fun when the ride to it has taken half an hour as when it has taken two hours.

A quite different type of holiday again is the one that offers a 'taste of riding' among other activities for the child or adult who has never ridden before. Here we are back to the enclosed space and all the help necessary for the complete beginner. Little can be achieved in so short a time, but some may go home wanting to 'ride properly' and with luck will have the chance later.

When going out on a ride extra attention should be given to correct fitting of saddlery and to provision of any extra items that may make for the comfort of rider and pony on a longer than usual expedition – neck straps to hang on to when going up steep hills, for example, and sheepskin saddle covers for some who may not need them at home. Girths require careful checking, especially before steep descents are made. Flies in high summer can be a menace from which there is no complete protection, but ample supplies of fly repellents (for the ponies) helps a bit! The leaders must be on constant lookout for hazards such as holes and loose wire, and riders should be taught to do the same. Narrow paths tend to give a sense of security, even when quite steep, and these are usually the places where leading reins can best be removed for the first time, although there must be constant reminders that to get on the heels of the pony in front is to run the risk of being kicked. It is when a party approaches a wide open space abreast that the competitive spirit in the ponies is apt to emerge, and the experienced leader will recognise the sparking points and take evasive action before any nonsense starts. The lunch break needs to be well managed, with the ponies safely tied up (by head collars, not reins). They too deserve their break. And once dismounted it must not be forgotten that everybody has to be got up again; a preliminary survey should be made for tree trunks etc., that can serve as mounting blocks – many a rider has discovered a new agility when faced with the necessity for making do without his usual convenient block. It is a wise precaution to make the picnic place one that can be reached by car or Land Rover, so that anyone really tired can be ferried home.

Attention to all these details, and careful planning of the routes, need not lessen the adventure quality of the holiday and are very necessary. How much of the day remains to be filled by other activities and outings will depend on the amount of time that can happily be spent riding. Those who have trekked for most of the day will not have a great deal of energy left, but those who are unable to ride for more than a short time will need organised occupations to fill the day. Swimming, when available, and in suitable weather, is always enjoyable after riding, and simple outings such as visits to farms usually give as much pleasure as ambitious sightseeing expeditions. The tendency is to forget just how long everything takes when there are a number of heavily handicapped people together; all too easily the day may be crammed so full that the essential relaxed atmosphere is lost. There should be time to make a social event of tack cleaning, for log books and diaries to be kept, for maps and bird books to be looked at and for that happy half hour leaning over the fence watching the resting ponies and talking over the day's excitements.

The Riding for the Disabled Association

The object of the Association is to give the opportunity of riding to disabled people who might benefit in their general health or well being.

Founded in 1969 and under the patronage of HRH The Princess Anne, this registered charity is an Association of Member Groups organised into seventeen administrative Regions in the British Isles. There are also a number of affiliated Overseas Groups and Associations. Privileges of membership include the provision of Insurance cover, access to training courses and Conferences, advisory services, and in certain cases financial assistance. Headquarters are a modest office building at Stoneleigh in Warwickshire where the Director, Secretary and a small staff are the only salaried personnel.

The general management of the Association is the responsibility of the Council on which each Region is represented and which has representatives from the medical and paramedical professions together with experts in other allied fields for formulating policies. These include the British Orthopaedic Association, British Paediatric Association, Chartered Society of Physiotherapy, British Association of Occupational Therapists, the Royal Society for Disability and Rehabilitation, the British Red Cross Society, the Spastics Society, the Sports Council, the National Council for Special Education, the British Horse Society, the British Veterinary Association and an Assessor appointed by the Department of Education and Science. Through its Standing Committees the Council can advise and assist Member Groups on such matters as finance, training, holidays, medical matters, the supply and welfare of horses and ponies and driving.

Each of the geographical Regions has an administrative committee which includes a Regional Instructor and an adviser from the Chartered Society of Physiotherapy.

Each of the Regions consists of a number of Counties and a County Representative is appointed in each one.

The vast majority of disabled children and adults who ride in this country do so in the care of Member Groups, of which there are in 1983 no less than 540 catering for some 17,340 riders, both physically and mentally handicapped, and also blind and deaf. These Groups vary from the very small to a few maintaining purpose-built centres which cater for several hundred riders each week. The ponies used may be owned by Groups, loaned by private owners, or hired from Riding Schools.

The Association has now built up a considerable fund of knowledge and experience, and anyone who may be contemplating the possibility of arranging riding for any handicapped people is urged to consider the advantages of Membership of the Association from whom they should seek advice.

A horse of your own?

Many a parent of a handicapped child, having heard about the virtues of riding, asks the question, 'Shall I buy him a pony?' And many an older rider who has found great fulfilment in riding feels the urge to plunge into ownership.

Sadly the answer to this question must usually be 'No'. The idea of the little pony as a substitute for pram or wheelchair does not usually work out well. The child is likely to become bored riding when only led out by his mother and will learn much more and find greater enjoyment riding with a group of other children. The pony reserved for one handicapped rider is likely to be under exercised and to become spoilt and naughty, and the fact must be faced that comparatively few people have the facilities for keeping a horse; once acquired it becomes a major responsibility. It must never be forgotten or neglected, and cannot be conveniently laid up like a motor bicycle. The expense of providing it with food, shoes and veterinary attention are considerable, and disability in the family often means that financial resources are strained. Stable work is hard work and that which starts as a pleasure can easily become a chore. It is irresponsible to take on ownership without facing up to the burdens that go with it.

As with everything else, however, there is always the exceptional case, the rider for whom nothing less than ownership will do. Provided he has learned to ride well enough to manage on his own without being a danger to himself and others, provided he is a responsible person who knows enough about the care of the animal, fully realises what is involved, and

can meet the needs one way or another, then who should say
'No' to him? He will certainly face extra problems, will need to
take great care and wise advice in finding a horse that suits him,
will probably need practical help from some source or another;
but for him there can be the special joy and fulfilment that
comes from having four good legs of his very own, a partner
with whom he can build up a relationship not available to the
once-a-week horseman.

There are different approaches to riding for the disabled and
various opinions as to how far it is a therapy, how far a
recreation. Possibly every handicapped rider finds in it
something slightly different, according to his needs and tastes.
What is indisputable is that it provides a stimulating challenge
that if taken up can bring the rewards of greater self
confidence, improved co-ordination and balance and great
enjoyment. An experienced physiotherapist has written,
'Evidence has shown that while there are many successful
techniques for mental stimulation and physical improvement,
the use of the horse is unrivalled as a means of achieving a
combination of both physical and mental benefits.' A disabled
rider has said, 'When I am on a horse I forget that I cannot
walk.' What more need be added?

6 Out on the hills

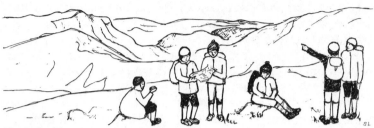

Introduction

For many handicapped people a walk in wild country might be their first taste of real adventure; a chance to experience large, open expanses of countryside – dark forests and damp moors, the rugged coast and remote mountains. What a difference from life in hospital or residential home with occasional visits to the city shops!

Rambling and hiking are among the most popular leisure activities in this country, enjoyed by millions each year. So why not the handicapped person? Often many difficulties will be raised by those responsible for arranging leisure programmes for disabled people: 'They wouldn't enjoy it' – 'Rather go shopping' – 'What about the wheelchairs?' – 'It may rain.' These, and many other comments are all too easily made – but what a pity. Our own experience is that with a more positive approach the wheelchair can be taken almost anywhere, and certainly over a greater range of terrain than is normally asked of it! Wheelchairs on cliffline coastal footpaths; along deep forest paths; across grass and heather moors; and even to the snow-beds of mountain peaks in the high Swiss Alps. Severity of handicap should not be a limiting factor, since adventure is in the mind of the participant and what is a thrill for the handicapped rambler may well seem tame for the helper.

For the mentally retarded young person the more traditional hike over the hills, in truly wild country, may be an ambition which can easily be realised, but young and old alike find great pleasure in their walks in open countryside. More particularly if the walk is of great interest rather than of great distance. A short two-mile hike, full of information about wildlife and plants, the local scenery and history, will be far more successful to the handicapped walker than ten miles at full pace, without much being known or said about the route. Countryside interpretation contributes much to our enjoyment.

Walks, rambles and hikes, in addition to providing pleasant leisure time, are also significant means of staying healthy. The overweight, rather lethargic young mentally handicapped individual is a common member of the population in training centres, hospital units and special schools. Diets are more successful when combined with a programme of exercise, and walking can be an enjoyable way of providing that exercise, while at the same time giving mental stimulation and educational opportunities. Health, excitement, learning all in *one* activity. This must be worth far more of our time!

In this chapter we shall not only explore the countryside on foot but also examine other means of transport, such as cycling. Much of the information on rambling applies equally well to other adventures, and many activities can be linked to environmental education and to short camp situations. We also take a look at orienteering and the possibilities for handicapped participants. Planning your own route, navigating your way through forests or across a desolate moor – these may appear at first thought to be impossible for most and not really worthy of consideration for those with intellectual limitations or confined to wheelchairs. But as we have seen earlier, everything is possible if we give it enough consideration. So let's take to the hills!

Hill walks and rambles

As with other adventure pursuits, it is important to progress slowly by a series of small steps, allowing participants to develop an interest in their newly found activity. There are many routes to follow between the town park and high moors and mountains. You may not wish to travel too far from home for your early hikes, but often there are good paths along disused railway lines or perhaps by the side of a river or canal.

Towpaths often provide attractive walks full of historic interest and with a wealth of wildlife. They serve major population areas and often give easy access to wheelchair users. Who knows? A walk by the side of the local canal may lead on to barge holidays or canoeing in weedy waters. The

Water Space Amenity Commission will supply a list of local Navigation Authorities, who will be able to tell you if waterways are open to walkers and whom to contact for permission. A long distance walk with a difference covers a hundred miles of Birmingham towpaths. The walk visits twelve canals and abounds with historic interest. Details are published in a guide *The Navigation Way* (Peter Groves; Tetradon Publications) – available from Bridge House, Shalford, Guildford.

Like towpaths, the old railway lines were flat, a very useful 'top priority' for those planning a wheelchair walk. They too are crowded with interesting plants and animals, some of which I described in my companion book in this series, *Out of Doors with Handicapped People*. Today there are thousands of miles of disused railway, some of them bought by Local Authorities and converted to amenity paths, often in 'areas of outstanding natural beauty'.

Many organisations will supply information packs with brochures and lists of good walks and rambles in your area. There are now over a hundred Country Parks within easy reach of roads and other services, including toilets, a list of which can be obtained from the offices of the Countryside Commission. Several have been laid out with trails and paths and take in a variety of good scenery and views, often within a short distance.

The National Trust owns and maintains much of our countryside, in addition to stately homes and gardens. Many coastal footpaths make delightful areas for rambling; wild flowers and seabirds provide constant interest and cliffs and dunes are ideal environments to create a real sense of adventure. The Trust provides excellent publicity information and your local office will give all necessary details.

Forest paths are always exciting, and with the growth of the Forestry Commission in post-war years we are now amply supplied with acres of dense plantations of pine, spruce and fir. The Commission has done much to open its forests to public use and they have rapidly learned the amenity value of their land. Many forests have good nature trails, picnic sites and toilets, and once again their information is excellent. Guide books and maps are available for many forest paths and nature trail booklets inform the readers about much of the wildlife living amongst the trees.

If you are fortunate, you may live close to one of our ten National Parks in England and Wales, which are much larger than the Country Parks and often encompass wild country. The Countryside Commission both in England and Scotland will send you a list of the parks, together with addresses of the local park office. Each park has a full-time warden and other staff who are only too keen to help you plan your route for a visit by disabled people. Indeed during the International Year of Disabled People in 1981 the Commission held a number of important conferences aimed at learning more about the requirements of handicapped people in the countryside, and especially in wild country. The results of these meetings, and of their own thoughts, have been published in an excellent report *Informal Countryside Recreation for Disabled People – Advisory Series No. 15* (The Countryside Commission).

Suggestions for rambling can often be found in the publications of the various Tourist Boards, and as well as routes to follow they supply information about interesting places you will find on the way. From the canals of the Midlands to the high peaks of Snowdonia, there are paths to follow and information abounds on them all.

It will be best if the leader can walk the route before making plans for his group, since this will confirm access details for any who use a wheelchair, any difficulties arising from path surfaces, availability of toilets and whether the route can be circular in nature rather than everyone having to return along the same path. If this is not possible it may be best to have transport waiting at the end of the hike, since a few miles spent on the main road after an interesting route has been followed can ruin the pleasure and excitement gained. The leader may like to take photographs of the route to show everyone, together with the published material available from the organisations mentioned.

The walk may be linked to a specific topic of interest – a list of flowers, trees or birds, a look at some historic buildings or a simple description of the scenery and landscape of the area. Projects always make for greater interest and will take minds off the distance still to be covered! I remember taking a group of mentally handicapped trainees, from a London Adult Training Centre, along what was to be a short coastal footpath hike. Almost immediately after our departure from the car park, along a rather muddy uphill stretch of narrow pathway, one young and overweight trainee remarked, 'Where's the bus stop?'

What to wear

Clearly the clothing most suitable for a hike along the canal bank is not always ideal for the high moors, and summer gear will not be adequate for winter in wild country. However, there are certain guidelines which, if followed, will remove many future problems. Cost will certainly be a major factor in any decision, especially when it comes to taking a group out rambling or hiking.

There is no purpose in specifying essential items, only for these to detract from the organisation of the activity itself. So, what will most people possess already and what is reasonable to expect them to purchase? In this country clothing is needed for warmth and waterproofing; remember that it is easier to remove items when one is too hot than it is to put on an extra layer which you did not bring! Several thin layers of clothes are also better insulation than one thick, heavy sweater or jacket. Wool is best, but man-made fibres will also be suitable fabric. While a light cotton or tee-shirt is suitable in summer, a woollen shirt or string vest will be better for winter or in wild country. Over this, wear two light sweaters for warmth and an anorak. This will provide a windproof layer so that the warm air trapped by your shirt and sweaters does not become disturbed by the cold air outside. Remember, warmth is provided by the retention of your own body heat. It cannot come from elsewhere.

Most people will possess a suitable anorak for normal use, usually with a full-length zip, but if you intend to purchase one, then a hood might be an added attraction. Other jackets or a parka could be worn if an anorak is not available. None of these garments, however, is waterproof and your final outside layer should be supplied in the form of a cagoule. If you need to buy one item of clothing it should be this one, and extra money is well worth spending at this stage. Look at the label and select a waterproof, not showerproof, garment. True, it will also

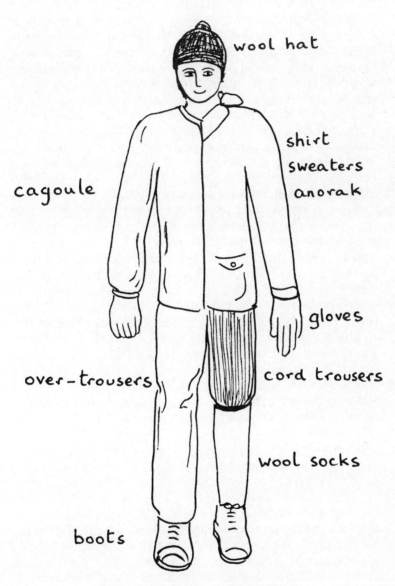

wool hat

shirt
sweaters
anorak

cagoule

gloves

over-trousers

cord trousers

wool socks

boots

Clothing for hiking in open country

retain moisture from within, but it is better to be slightly damp from your own sweat than to be soaked by a heavy downpour of rain. You do not need to walk all the time in your cagoule but it should be handy for the sudden shower. A pair of over-trousers would be a good idea at the same time and are very cheap to buy. They will save your trousers from getting wet from rain running down over the cagoule onto your legs, as well as from the damp vegetation you may have to walk through. Life can be quite pleasant inside a waterproof cagoule and trousers even when the sky is black, a wind is blowing and the rain lashes down from above! That's not to say you should begin your adventure in such conditions but at the same time it may well happen before you return.

Your other clothes should be readily available. Cord trousers are generally considered better than jeans, which when wet are very uncomfortable, cling to the legs and take a long time to dry out. But if you are not going far, or are travelling in lowland areas, then jeans will be quite suitable. Females should wear the same style of clothing as the males; thin cotton dresses and skirts are not at all appropriate for hiking on the moors or for negotiating that stile along the canal path. Headgear is equally important and a woolly hat can be worn at most times since considerable heat is lost via the head. Gloves, too, should be carried since many find their hands quickly become cooled, especially when wet; this can lead to misery.

Those individuals who are not active and require a wheelchair must certainly have gloves available, but their other clothes are as for other people. Instead of an anorak a waterproof cycle cape can be ideal for the wheelchair user and extra warmth to the legs can be supplied by a special quilted covering designed by certain manufacturers for this purpose. For the handicapped person we find footwear can be the biggest single problem of clothing. The wheelchair user can continue to wear normal heavy shoes but the physically handicapped walker often has enough foot problems without making special demands for hiking needs. Under such circumstances one can only say that shoes need to be strong, comfortable and as waterproof as possible. Dubbin will help in this respect and a 'before and after' treatment will give better results than neglect.

What suits one person will not necessarily be best for another. Light shoes or trainers are often good enough for summer weather walking in easy country and rubber welling-tons, although often looked upon with scorn by hikers, can be suitable in muddy conditions or on wet moorland hikes which are not too long. They are not suitable on rocky surfaces and where they will slip, but for many of your walks they are often appropriate. Good heavy-duty wool socks are essential with wellingtons, giving warmth and comfort. Even newspaper layers in the boot will act in this capacity and soon become worn into the shape of the foot. Your thick boot socks should be worn over an ordinary pair of wool socks and remember that good foot care can often be best provided by attention to your socks. Nylon socks should be avoided since feet sweat and they do not allow air to circulate next to the skin.

Hiking boots will seldom be in the possession of handicapped people and good boots are costly. But do not let this deter you from going out on that hike, since many able-bodied people *prefer* to walk in ordinary footwear. If boots are to be bought you will have a wide choice from shoe shops, stores (Army & Navy, Millets . . .) and specialist sports gear shops. Prices will show an enormous range and generally you get what you pay for. Select for comfort a pair of boots which appear pliable. Hard rigid heels which rub ankles can easily finish the hike after very few miles. Take heavy-duty socks with you when buying boots and allow a little space in the boot for foot expansion when selecting the correct size. Wear them in gently in the house for a few days before venturing outdoors. This way you can change them if you find they are unsuitable. Your first walks must be short and gentle, since boots take considerable time to mould to the shape of your feet.

What shall I carry?
Anything you think you may require or wish to take on the hike is best carried in a small rucksack or day-pack, leaving hands free and giving you better balance. For the day out on a quiet walk you will not need to take much but on a longer hike in winter, or in wild areas, the list becomes longer and reaches an ultimate level for the backpacker. Many chainstores will sell you a nylon day-pack which is adequate enough to hold your

waterproofs, some food and drink and a few other desirable items of equipment. Everything is best packed inside a large polythene bag, such as a dustbin liner, since your rucksack will not be waterproof. Place your waterproofs near the top or at the back of the pack, so that they form a flat, softer layer against your own back. Avoid awkward shapes which dig into your body. Some items can be carried in your pockets – matches, a penknife, a pencil and notepad, string, some toilet paper, sun glasses, a can/bottle opener, the maps and compass. Wear a watch or make sure your companions have one.

The group leader at least should carry a first aid kit on all walks, wherever you go or at whatever time of year. The kit can be kept in a small tin or polythene box (a plastic food box is ideal). It should contain basic items such as a variety of strip plasters; roll of bandage; 3mm crepe bandage; Melolin gauze dressings; antiseptic cream; antihistamine cream; Paracetamol or similar headache tablets; suncream; scissors. If you are taking a group of handicapped people, obviously check on individual medical requirements and carry with you any drugs and medicine required – there will usually be several!

Particular care should be taken with 'hidden handicaps' such as epilepsy and diabetes. In the case of diabetics remember that exertion above normal uses up food reserves (blood sugar) much quicker than might be expected and frequent eating of biscuits and other easily digested foodstuffs might be necessary. Over-tiring should be avoided and keep a constant watch for signs of fatigue which may lead to a coma.

In general, foods for a day's hike should have high energy content, be pleasant and easy to eat and preferably light to carry. In winter, and indeed at most other seasons, hot soup in a vacuum flask makes even the dullest sandwiches taste good, and forms ideal food and liquid in a single meal. Cake, biscuits, chocolate, nuts and dried fruit are all suitable high energy foods giving a rapid intake of calories which will be utilised for your extra exertions and lost in heat production. Such foods are also good morale boosters and eating should be little and often. A large mid-day meal and rest is undesirable since you will not want to start walking again afterwards. Lethargy soon sets in – you will feel sleepy and find the homeward trek quite a struggle. Also the heat generated by your body is soon lost in sweating when you stop to rest and the first sign of this is a sudden involuntary shivering while you are sitting down or standing still. To avoid this put on an extra layer of clothing, if you have one in your pack, move about a little rather than sitting all the time and keep your rest periods short and frequent. A piece of chocolate every half-hour is a far better incentive and better nutritionally, than eating the whole bar at one sitting. Liquid is heavy to carry and should be considered as a provider of energy, as well as water to the body. Fruit, such as apples and oranges are compact ways in which to carry your liquid.

Adventurous rambles

You will soon find that lowland country paths, canal banks and bridleways cease to provide the challenge that awaits you further afield. In most parts of Britain large tracts of open country are within easy reach: the Downs and Wealds of south-east England; the Chilterns, Mendips and Cotswolds; the south-west coastal footpath – you need not live close to mountainous regions to find good, adventurous walking. However, much of our wild country is set in west or northern Britain – Dartmoor, Snowdonia, the Lake District and the Highlands of Scotland.

Fortunately centres of high population and many conurbations are equally close to remote, exciting landscapes. Manchester and Sheffield are within an hour of the Peak district, many Yorkshire and Lancashire towns lie close to the high hills of the Pennine chain and Birmingham walkers can escape to the routes of Cannock Chase and the Malverns. Nowhere do we have far to travel in order to find long hikes in adventurous surroundings. Many of the books listed in the Appendix give full details of routes for different parts of the country with information about distances, maps and access. Some parts will be suitable for a single day's outing, but others will necessitate a weekend or even a walking holiday. This is certainly true for the official long-distance routes which are marked by the famous 'acorn' emblem and administered by The Countryside Commission. Many are very long, arduous undertakings for even the 'professional' walker. Don't tackle the 250 miles of the Pennine Way until you have tried several of the much shorter unofficial routes which may be only twenty to thirty miles of easier terrain.

London-based ramblers are fortunate to have more of these routes within easy reach than any other part of the country. The 'London Countryway' is a circular path, about 15–30 miles from the City, with bus and train links for one day or weekend hiking. A guide is published (*A Guide to the London Countryway*, B.K.Chesterton, Constable). The total route is over 200 miles long and gives plenty of options. 'The North Downs Way' follows roughly the Pilgrim's Way along the line of the North Downs through Surrey and Kent. It keeps to the crest of the hills for 141 miles, with fine views to the south. Once again a guide is published.

If you are intent on trying a weekend of walking then accommodation overnight will be a major consideration unless you intend to backpack and carry tent, sleeping bag and other essential equipment, thus necessitating a much larger and heavier rucksack. Most hikers and other form of travellers use the hostels of the YHA for single nights, since they are inexpensive and the network covers most quarters of the countryside. A full list of addresses and a guide on how to find each of them is supplied to members of the Association and you can join at the hostel on your first night. But check that accommodation is available, particularly in busy seasons.

Clearly if you are planning to organise an overnight hike which involves wheelchair users then special arrangements may be necessary. Again travel the route first before taking others along and look out for ideas on accommodation (church or village halls, community centres, schools, a farm barn) as well as studying access problems and path surfaces. Some routes will be perfectly satisfactory – others will not! In certain situations you may need to take sleeping bags and foam bedrolls along before your hike, and plan the catering arrangements if you are not staying in a hostel or in similar accommodation. Your local Tourist Board office may be able to help.

Walking in wild country
While all that has been said earlier about rambling and hiking applies equally well, irrespective of the countryside in which

you are venturing, there are certain added precautions necessary if you are planning an adventure in winter or on wild desolate moors and mountains.

Firstly, watch the weather. Remember that weather differs at high altitudes from down in the town or valley, and can change rapidly. Often deterioration in conditions will occur from early morning as the day progresses. Always obtain an up-to-date weather forecast for the locality in which you are going to hike. The television weather programme from the night before is certainly not sufficient. Telephone a local services camp or station, Mountain Rescue centre, Meteorological station and, if you are still uncertain, the local police station.

Inform some authority, such as the police, of your route, expected time of arrival back at base and number of walkers. Always remember to inform them as soon as you return, to safeguard against unnecessary concern for your welfare. Never underestimate the weather or mountainous countryside. If you feel the conditions are too arduous, or that deterioration is likely, while you are in wild country, then begin your return immediately. Do not venture further with hopes of improvement in conditions. They seldom occur and the time wasted can be significant in the safe return of your party to base. High winds; heavy driving rain; sleet and hail; thick mists; cold temperatures; snow . . . all of these conditions can suddenly appear and are enough to hasten your departure from the hills. As conditions worsen it will take you longer to get back, morale rapidly lowers and problems emerge for the leader.

Safety in wild country cannot be stressed too strongly. Your walking clothing must be adequate and footwear suitable for rough terrain. Plenty of warm layers should provide insulation and gloves and hat are essential for everybody.

The leader must carry additional safety equipment in a strong framed rucksack. This should include a sleeping bag or Bivi-bag, a survival bag of strong polythene, into which anyone can be placed suffering from exposure problems or following an accident. Aluminium foil, thermal blankets take up very little space and are of low weight, and can be useful to wrap individuals in exposure conditions.

Emergency rations are also a must on the list. They should be high in energy content – chocolate, nuts and raisins, Kendal mint cake, glucose tablets, barley sugar. In addition, a meal of dehydrated food can be easily carried for the group, together with a small Gaz burner and lightweight aluminium cooking utensil. Drinks are readily prepared from Oxo cubes, jar of Marmite or Bovril, and similar standard preparations, which can be dissolved in water from a stream (or even melted snow). Such items should be a permanent feature of the survival pack, along with a whistle, torch and first aid kit. Many leaders will feel they should also carry a rope attached to their pack which can be used to make a rescue from cliffs, mountain crags, a river or other feature of the landscape.

While maps and compass ought to feature on *all* your walks, it is of vital importance that they accompany the hiker in wild country and that an experienced leader should be able to use them to navigate a route across unknown terrain in bad conditions. A descending mist can fall in minutes, obscuring landmarks and giving a completely false impression of direction. Under such circumstances a map and compass are your only hope of returning home safely.

Leaders can obtain training at specialist outdoor centres and may consider the Mountain Leadership Certificate (MLC), courses for which are conducted at centres such as Plas y Brenin in Snowdonia which is administered by the Sports Council. Additional expertise may be obtained from local organisers of the Duke of Edinburgh Award Scheme, County Youth Services, Scout and Guide leaders, teachers in Outdoor Pursuits, Wardens of Outward Bound and similar centres. Such organisations may also be willing to assist with loaning equipment for anyone wishing to take handicapped people into wild country.

In the event of an accident or other such emergency it is desirable to return to safe ground and base as soon as possible, but under some circumstances this may not be possible. Serious injury to a member of the party may necessitate one staff member returning alone for assistance leaving behind the injured individual with another staff member. This situation illustrates the importance of high staff ratios in organising excursions with handicapped participants.

Those remaining behind should be left as safe as possible, in comfortable surroundings, with warmth and food. The injured person should be placed in the sleeping bag or survival bag, in full clothing. Shelter from bad weather conditions can be supplied by natural ground features such as large boulders, a small cave, a wall or anything else to reduce the effects of wind and driving rain, snow or hail. Collect anything that will give some insulation from the ground – bracken fern is ideal – and if time allows construct a bivouac shelter using a large polythene sheet kept down at the edges by stones and rocks. Tree branches, gorse and old heather bushes can all be used if a polythene sheet is not available. However, for its weight and the space it will occupy, such a useful piece of luggage can be placed at the bottom of any leader's rucksack.

Make sure you know the return route and exact location where the injured party has been left, especially in thick mists and deteriorating conditions. Check times and note how long it takes to reach help and make an emergency telephone call to the police. This will assist when you are making the return journey; only leave someone behind if you are certain that to proceed further will increase the severity of the injury, or that the delay in time might endanger everyone else in the group.

To summarise, it is important to follow these six basic principles of first aid in the event of accidents and injury when in wild country:

1   Prevent further injury and if necessary move patient to a safe place if there is likely to be further danger from his present position.
2   Maintain breathing and circulation which may necessitate mouth to mouth resuscitation. Practise beforehand under the instruction of a qualified person.
3   Stop bleeding, usually by direct pressure with the hand or a pad.
4   Treat for shock – keep the patient warm in a resting position, providing extra shelter if necessary and possible. Hot, sweet drinks may be sipped. It is not desirable to give alcohol.
5   Seek help – write down all details on the accident and give the exact position wherever possible (map reference). Provide information about the casualty. Take considerable care in seeking help – two injured persons will not help the circumstances.

6   Evacuate if worsening conditions make it likely that the patient will have the best chance by being taken from the scene of the accident.

However it is best not to place yourself in this situation and careful planning can help to eliminate all but the most unfortunate of emergencies.

Orienteering

While true orienteering is often undertaken competitively at a fast pace against the stopwatch, we have found that an adapted form of this activity provides a suitable adventure pursuit for both mentally and physically handicapped youngsters.

For most orienteers the map and compass are essential pieces of equipment, but although their use is described later in this chapter it proves far too difficult for many handicapped participants. Consequently, in an effort to find a suitable navigation system, especially in wild country, for use by those who are mentally retarded or have learning difficulties, we have introduced a photographic system.

First a suitable course is selected, often over an area of moorland without obvious footpaths and featuring a variety of interesting land features. The route is then walked by staff and the distance checked as being suitable for the participants. Two or three miles is an ideal distance for introducing such an orienteering activity. Photographs are taken at strategic points along the course: a stream to be crossed; a boggy area to be watched; a rocky outcrop for climbing over; a stone wall or fence where you change direction; a lone tree or bush which makes an obvious landmark; the end-point of the course which should be easily identifiable (for example, a lake, car park, public house).

Photographs can be taken in black and white, enlarged and presented to the group, or colour prints from an Instamatic or a Polaroid camera could also be found suitable. They should be numbered according to the route to be followed and annotated if necessary with comments such as 'turn right here'; 'take care – wet ground'; 'go through this gate'; 'climb this rocky area'; 'stop walking here'. The 'photo-pack' can be shown to the participants beforehand, but after several routes have been followed it may be possible to give them a new course and 'photopack' which is unseen.

The group should follow their course in small groups or in pairs and cope with decisions regarding direction and terrain by themselves. Staff can be placed at the beginning and end of the course and at strategic points along a route, where they can observe the activity without participants relying on their involvement. In this way safety aspects can be observed, no one need get lost and yet the handicapped orienteers make all decisions. We have found that often the most unlikely candidates succeed and show an ability to organise and lead others.

Physically disabled participants often undertake quite arduous aspects of the course under their own initiative. For example, an athetoid, adolescent student, limited in walking and using arm crutches, not only completed a tough course in November over Bodmin Moor but in addition decided to climb the peak of a rocky tor which could very easily have been by-passed around the base. At the end of the course, having negotiated wet boggy areas, streams and rocky ground under cold winter conditions, with hail and sleet in the wind, he arrived at the car park with arms raised and crutches aloft in a triumphant gesture! Success that morning had been his.

A similar system can be devised for wheelchair orienteers, although thought must be given to problems of access; in this respect the land managed by the Forestry Commission is of particular value since there are frequently routes through dense conifer woodland which are maintained by them in the event of fire. An approach to the local office of the Forestry Commission should give you approval to investigate a suitable course, and often the Commission will arrange for gates to be unlocked if you require access for a vehicle. Clearly you may find similar co-operation in your own area with other official bodies, such as the National Trust, or with private land owners. The 'photopack' can be prepared in much the same way, although forests tend to lack such obvious landmarks as we find on moors. One might say that 'one tree looks just like another!' At difficult points a temporary marker might indicate the route. A map can also be made with appropriate distances along the tracks and turnings clearly marked. This can be linked to simple compass work if possible and makes a good way to teach aspects of geography. The map can be mounted on board under polythene and a copy given to each participant.

Most wheelchair users will require someone to push them along forest paths which, while substantial, are not good enough for self-propulsion. Gradients in some parts may be too steep for the handicapped orienteer to get himself along without assistance. Where do we get such helpers? Frequently you will find a local school where teachers (and pupils) are only too keen to become involved since it is considered good social development for the children and they too can participate in the outdoor activity. At weekends, or during holidays, it is possible to involve clubs (PHAB, Youth, Church), Scouts and Girl Guides, and even to match ages of children to some extent. In the event of such helpers being involved they should be taught to allow their wheelchair partner to make decisions on routes and directions and not to leave everything to the 'pusher'. It should develop into a real partnership rather than be one-directional.

Orienteer courses can also be designed for other forms of transport, especially for the person who cannot walk easily. A horserider can very easily participate in such a course over a wide variety of landscapes which might prove impossible for the wheelchair user. Similarly, on water the use of canoes would be ideal for orienteering about a river system which gave access to several creeks, or perhaps in a lake or reservoir. Markers could point the direction to the next point and maps are easily constructed to cover any type of course and terrain.

While thinking about the nature of maps, it is of interest to find that in Norway blind participants frequently orienteer on traditional forest courses. This activity is well described by Inge Morisbak, from the Beitostolen Centre, in an article presented in the Bradford Papers (1982). The map is tactile and constructed on plywood, with a ground plan outlined. Houses are small pieces of plywood glued in position; roads are 5mm strips of sandpaper of varying textures; grainy papers are paved roads and heavily grained indicates dirt roads. Stitched nylon traces at intervals along the roads show distances. Streams are plastic strings glued in position and fences are marked by pins placed in the baseboard. Small pins pressed fully down show the places where the post-markers are sited and similar pins on one side of the road in a road crossing indicate which side you should go. To find the post-marker a bearing system (sender and receiver) is used. The sender is placed as a post-marker, beeping signals with different frequencies in 360°. An ear-plug is attached to the receiver and the orienteer turns with the receiver. The direction with the lowest signals in its direction is from the sender or post-marker. A rope guides the orienteer towards the post and back to the road. While a helper is used in the first attempt at the course the aim is to do it independently. 'Through the combined use of the tactile sense by feeling the map with the hands and the ground with the feet, and the use of the auditive sense by using the bearing equipment and listening to nature's own sounds (eg running streams, echo) orienteering is found to be an exciting activity for the blind.'

Map and compass

Most ramblers, hikers, cyclists and outdoor fanatics are acquainted with the Ordnance Survey (OS) maps, and in particular with the new series of Landranger maps (scale 1:50,000). These replaced the older style 'one-inch' maps, although many will still be using these for years to come. On the new scale 2cm represent 1 kilometre (= 0.6214 miles), so that the nearest equivalent is that 3cm approximately represents 1 mile. It may however be best to think in terms of kilometres when you travel.

In certain localities you will be able to purchase special maps covering specific districts of exceptional interest (the Lake District, Dartmoor, the Cairngorms). These Outdoor Leisure Maps are printed on the 1:25,000 scale as are the new Pathfinder maps, which means 4cm represent 1 kilometre and greater detail, such as field boundaries, can be presented. A key to the meaning of symbols is given at the side of the map and these should become familiar to leaders and all walkers who will appreciate their significance.

A great deal of information can be gleaned from study of a map, including the shape of the ground or relief. This is indicated on the map by contour lines, marked in brown and spaced at 10 metre intervals. In addition to showing the height above sea-level of the land, the contours are closer together as the slope of the ground increases. Thus, several contour lines grouped closely together and rising to a summit height indicate you will be climbing steeply on your hike. Widely spaced contours obviously show a shallow gradient. The summit heights are given in metres, so that land over 2000 feet will be marked at approximately 700 metres.

Learn land relief by observing the contour lines when you are walking; it will make route planning easier on future trips. In addition, a better understanding of your map will make for more accurate navigation and recognition of your position in open country. Hills, woods, peaks, rivers, quarries, marshy ground . . . all are marked and may be important features to observe on your hike.

Safety is often dependent on how well you can read your map and use your compass which is useful in lowlands and essential in the hills. It can be used for both direction finding and to tell you how to reach a point in misty conditions when the map alone is of limited use.

Although there are many makes of compass, it is generally accepted that the Silva design is very suitable for hiking, orienteering and for most other activities and is easy to use. The compass can first be used to set your map, relating the map symbols to the actual details on the ground, so that the church is in the correct place relative to the stream you must cross and the wood which should be on your right. Turn the compass dial so that 'north' coincides with the direction-of-travel arrow on the transparent base plate. Position the compass on the map so that the edge of the base plate lies along any N-S grid line on the map. Now, without moving the compass, turn the map until the red point of the needle sits at the 352° mark on the rim. Use this degree mark, rather than 360°, to allow for the variation between grid north on the map and compass magnetic north. The map is now set and features on the map are directly relatable to the terrain. Go outside into the garden or park and simply try it yourself!

Now let's try to identify a particular feature. The church tower in the distance could be one of several shown on the map . . . but which? Point the direction-of-travel arrow at the feature and rotate the dial until the red end of the needle points to 352°. Place the compass on the map, so that the base plate edge just touches your own position. Rotate the compass until N on the dial points to the top of the map and the red orienting lines on the base should be parallel with the N-S grid lines on the map. The church will now lie on the edge of the compass or on a line extending from it.

If you are uncertain of your precise position on the map but you have been following a path, stream, valley or other line feature, this technique can be used in reverse. Identify a feature, which is represented on the map, at roughly right angles to you. Point the compass at the feature, turn the dial until the needle points to 352° and place the edge of the compass base-plate on the map to touch the feature sighted upon. Rotate the whole compass until the orienting lines are parallel to the grid lines. The point at which the base-plate edge cuts across the line feature you are travelling is your exact position. You can then proceed to identify other landmarks around you.

Sometimes the route you are following, perhaps a footpath, is marked on the map but suddenly disappears as an obvious landmark. You know your position but are not certain how to follow this disappearing path! Once again, lay your compass on the map, with the edge of the base-plate along the line of the footpath and the direction-of-travel arrow pointing from your position towards the route you wish to follow. Turn the dial so that N points to the top of the map and the orienting lines are parallel with the grid lines. The angle between N and the travel arrow is your bearing and you have used the compass as a protractor. Remove the compass from the map and turn it to coincide the red end of the needle with N. The travel arrow now points the way which you must go if you are to follow the disappearing path.

If you are following a bearing and wish to return along the same route, leave the compass dial alone but turn the whole compass until the white end of the needle points to N (or 352° if your bearing was taken from a map). Similarly, the compass can be used alone, without the map, to guide you towards a prominent feature, such as a mountain, when you cannot obviously see your route. Once again the travel arrow is pointed at the feature, the dial turned to coincide the red end of the arrow with N on the rim and after following the line of the travel arrow for a short distance you should re-establish this direction.

Cycling

Wheels can often give a great deal of independent mobility to physically disabled people. Young and old alike are able to explore the roads for distances which might be quite impossible on foot. Luggage can be carried more easily than when it has to be in a rucksack on your back, and the cycle camper has a degree of independence not often associated with disability.

Wheels come in a variety of forms, and while conventional bicycles can be ridden by many people with a significant handicap, we should also think about the use of both tandems and tricycles. The tandem enables the blind or partially sighted cyclist actively to partake in the activity behind a sighted rider, and tricycles are often used in schools by many physically handicapped youngsters, especially those who can walk but with only a limited degree of co-ordination. For them the tricycle becomes an essential part of normal life and its use can easily be extended from a mere visit to the local shops to full touring capacity.

Planning a cycle tour can be great fun – it may involve a single day's excursion into the local countryside; a one night cycle camp, either in tents or at a Youth Hostel; or a full tour over many miles involving more equipment, planning and adventure. Clearly a gradual approach is again to be recommended – muscles are used which previously one didn't realise existed and the sore posterior is well known to the long-distance cyclist! Find out initially just how far *you* can comfortably travel in a day and use this as your guide for touring. If you intend to cycle over several days then reduce your travel distance to allow for tiring. You may be able to cycle ten miles without effort in one day, but will you continually repeat this distance each day for a week?

Plan your route if possible to avoid long steep hills, although this may be impossible and you will just have to think of pushing up (or down) some of them. Think about your meals carefully and perhaps ensure that each day you pass through a town or large village to purchase your day's supplies. This will mean less weight to carry on the journey. Allow some rest days in your itinerary for sight-seeing and leave time to see things and places each day. There is no fun being in the saddle all the time.

What do you need to take? Essentially the gear of the cycle camper is that of the back-packer, with the similar provision that it depends on where you plan to spend the nights. Your supplies should be carried in pannier bags attached to a carrier frame at the rear of the bicycle. Across the top of the two panniers can be the tent roll, tent poles and sleeping mat – assuming you intend to camp. The panniers should be balanced for weight and those items required first near the top. Isolate your cooking utensils and light-weight stove away from food and clothes. A cycle cape is cheap to buy and best to keep you waterproof. It can be fixed alongside your tent roll. Luggage must be secure – use good leather straps or a 'spring-octopus' fixing device. Most equipment needed – panniers, frame, fixers – can be purchased from the retail cycle shops.

The standard wire basket attached to the rear of the tricycle may give sufficient room to pack all necessary items, which could be retained in large polythene bags or even in a suitable rucksack. At no time should rucksacks be carried on your back by the cyclist. Tentage and other large equipment will fix easily on top of the wire basket with straps. Some further items, such as daily food purchases, could be carried in the front basket if one is present. The key is clearly adaptability with safety: do not overload; take what is necessary; balance your load; carry things on the cycle rather than on you. Remember to check your brakes when the cycle is fully loaded, as the weight carried increases your momentum and thus the stopping distance.

So many things can be seen by the cyclist that in many ways it is the best of the touring methods. The hard physical side of hiking and backpacking is removed, the heavier items necessary for camping are taken by the cycle, distances travelled can be greater and thus the area of interest is extended and yet the pace of travel is slow enough for you still to 'use your eyes'. Landscape, wildlife, history are all combined with that spirit of adventure.

7 Going to camp

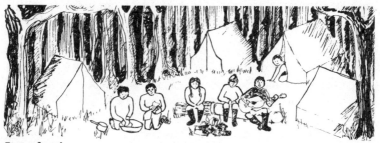

Introduction

Sleeping out-of-doors under a roof of canvas can be an adventure all by itself. Crawling in and out of the tent on all-fours; the smell of crackling bacon first thing in the morning; the welcome warmth of the sleeping bag again at night, are all part of the unique experience of camping. Yet there are still surprisingly many handicapped people who have never had the opportunity to partake in such a simple activity. One might suggest that no one is too handicapped to go to camp, providing the system is made as adaptable as necessary. True, there are many grades of camping, from the luxury of the caravan or large frame tent, complete with several rooms, to the lightweight nylon shelter of the 'wild camper'.

As with all other activities, it is important to begin simply and concentrate on life in an outdoor environment, for there is no better time to introduce the natural world to either retarded or disabled people. At first light the dawn chorus begins to arouse the sleeping camper, the sun rises to warm through the tent, giving an orange glow and often a false impression of just how bright it really is outside. During the day you are in constant contact with the sights, sounds and smells of the countryside, irrespective of where you camp. Even on the edge of a large city camp sites are remarkably rural, often in large park or forest locations. There may be a sighting of deer and at least some squirrels. Birds appear from high above to feed near the tent on scraps from an earlier meal. Many birds become amazingly tame when in contact with people – and their food – and will even sit on your hand to take crumbs of bread. As night draws in the birds move to roost, an owl gives a weird shriek and a hedgehog snuffles behind the tent. It is time for bed, there's a damp feeling in the air and as you lie on the ground warm and content the patter of rain falls against the tent. For it is not always dry and sunny at camp! But tomorrow is another day – and there will be more activity and plenty to be done again.

In the following pages we shall describe some of the skills of camping, which form such an important basis of many other activities. The hiker becomes a backpacker, the cyclist a cycle camper, the canoeist a canoe camper . . . for there are many ways to travel to camp. All will have similar needs, including somewhere to sleep and cook a meal, especially when low costs must be borne in mind. We learn about camp sites and tents, sleeping bags and bed rolls, cooking stoves and wood fires, camp food and meals. Camping may be a one-day or one-week experience, near to home or far away, and later we shall see how full-scale expeditions can be organised for handicapped participants. There is as much enjoyment to be gained from planning a camp, or expedition, as in actually taking part, and wherever possible everyone should be involved in these early stages. Looking at the maps, deciding on the venue, listing and checking the gear, buying supplies and making menus are all part of the trip. Let's away to camp and have fun!

Camping adventure

Perhaps we shall decide that our initial camp experience will be near to home and over a weekend. The group have not been to camp before – there are only six of them, but two boys are normally in wheelchairs and all require considerable help. Camping is for all ages, so our group could be a young family, children from the special school, young trainees from the local Adult Training Centre or much older residents from one ward of a long-stay hospital. In fact all such handicapped persons have spent one or two nights under canvas during an activity week at our outdoor education centre in Cornwall – and all have enjoyed it immensely. But where shall we take our six? How many helpers are required? What about tents and other equipment? Where shall we go to borrow things? Is there anything else that we have forgotten?

Many local inhabitants are often only too happy to assist in providing a camp site. If you have a permanent site close by, or farmers who provide temporary camping ground, then this might be the best start. There are many facilities which could be useful, especially wash-rooms and toilets. Visit the site beforehand and check access for your wheelchairs, but be prepared to adapt attitudes to narrow doorways, small toilet areas, cold water and anything else you may not find in the school or hospital. Often the permanent site is best if you are taking a severely handicapped group and I have personally selected such a situation for a foreign expedition.

However, if the campers are more mobile, active and capable of 'rougher' treatment then search for a more remote site. Check farmers, Forestry Commission or private woodland, owners of large estates with parkland and ask permission to camp with your small group. Again visit the site with the owner and confirm access details, water supply, toilet arrangements and any supply of fresh foods, such as milk and eggs. These are not necessary but can make life enjoyable. It is also fun for your campers to make the morning walk to the farm, bringing back warm eggs fresh from beneath the hens (perhaps having even collected them) and milk which is not in bottles and smells different. Camping can be highly educational! They may be able to collect firewood from beneath the local forest trees and will surely want to cook meals over an open wood fire and sit around the campfire that evening to sing songs. Confirm with the owner that such an open fire is allowed, not a risk to local timbers and where it can be sited.

So we have found a location to camp – what next? How many will be going and how many tents are required? You always need more helpers than you originally felt necessary. It is almost the case that you think of a number and double it! If the six all need some care assistance – dressing and undressing, washing, help with toilet and two have to be pushed in wheelchairs, I would always take six staff over a long-stay camp. Perhaps on a weekend only you could do with four, but it is better to have too many than too few. It is a very long day and much time in camp is spent in surviving. It takes far more time just to do everything – water fetching, cooking, washing up, personal hygiene, changing clothes, lighting the fire, collecting fuel . . . the day soon goes. Add to this the hours spent in care assistance and remember that you are working under much more difficult conditions. Dressing two boys inside a tent – removing the sleeping bag, searching for the right trouser leg, pulling them on and fastening a zip and belt in the horizontal situation – does not make for an easy life. So rather than staying at home, take extra helpers.

Camp equipment
Tents vary a great deal and choice may depend on what you have available or can borrow. You may approach the County Youth Service, who have considerable access to equipment, or the local Scout or Guide Movement. A small frame tent will give greater height to work with the boys who use wheelchairs, and the outer compartment is ideal for changing clothes and housing the empty chairs at night. During the day this outer area may be suitable for other care duties or for eating a meal if the weather is cold or wet. Tentage for the others will depend on the sex ratio, but if we assume two boys and two girls, then we shall require two small ridge tents. If they are all of the same sex, then a 4-man ridge tent would be suitable. There are many good manufacturers, but we have found Vango to be ideal, especially for wheelchair campers, since you can purchase an extension piece which fits onto the front opening and is convenient storage space for wheelchairs, arm crutches, other aids and personal luggage.

For comfortable camping if weight is not important, a mess tent should be taken, comprising an extensive area of canvas roof held from a ridge pole by guy ropes, but with open sides and ends. The Army uses them when in camp and could loan one for your weekend. They are ideal for eating under, cooking in mud or rain, wet days, evening activities . . . and even writing postcards to Mum and Dad! On expeditions they serve a multipurpose role which adds significantly to both comfort and efficiency.

You will of course require tents for the helpers, and while one big one may seem easier, three smaller ones will give more privacy and create a more harmonious camp. In terms of weight there is probably little difference and the latter system may well be lighter due to the materials used (nylon rather than canvas; aluminium poles and not wood).

We now need sleeping bags and something to sleep on. Most

modern tents have sewn-in ground sheets, but if not you will have to plan on separate waterproof ones. The simplest sleeping rolls are made from polythene foam or a similar material which has a porous nature. The air trapped forms the insulating layer between the ground and the body. Camping mats are cheap, easy to carry and ideal for backpacking or lightweight camping. Other alternatives are airbeds, which must be pumped-up 'in situ', or camp beds. The handicapped camper may need 'a cushion effect', especially if pressure sores easily develop and air beds may then be best. Take a foot pump, spare stoppers and a repair kit. Accidents easily happen – usually in the middle of the night when leaks suddenly appear from nowhere! Camp beds are of course bulky items to carry but may be suitable for the older or severely physically disabled camper. Tents will need to be larger in area and height if camp beds are used.

Bedding is seldom taken to camp since a sleeping bag is usually simpler and very warm. Bags are mostly terylene-filled, although down feathers provide insulation in the best bags and modern manufacturers use holo-fil. The latter have the advantage that if they get wet they retain their insulating properties. Some bags have full-length zips which are often convenient for physically disabled campers; they can be laid down flat on the open bag and simply zipped in position. Short length zips or tie-neck openings are preferred by many since no heat is lost via the long zip. If sleeping bags cannot be bought or borrowed then blankets will have to suffice – which in summer need present no problems. Large blanket pins, or even nappy pins, will hold the edges of a folded blanket in position to make an improvised sleeping bag. An unfolded blanket tends to fall away in the night leaving a cold sleeper! Several blankets will need to be used or a duvet can be wrapped over the person once inside the blanket bag.

While one may feel too warm on entering a sleeping bag it becomes much colder during the night and early hours of the morning, so a light sweater or sweatshirt should be worn over pyjamas. Socks too may help prevent cold feet. Girls should dress similarly, for if you are not warm in the night it is unlikely that you will sleep.

Camp planning should include cooking and eating. Do we

take a table and chairs? What type of stove should we use? What about utensils? Visitors to other European countries often remark that the camping scene is very civilised, organised and comfortable. Families spend several weeks under canvas, and often seem to have removed their house contents to the country or coast. Seldom do you see them all sitting on the grass, eating off plates perched precariously on knees, with the stove and washing up bowl at ground level. But perhaps this is not true camping? The answer clearly is that you should live in the manner which suits you best. Certainly a folding metal camping table and folding camp chairs are not costly to buy in the large chain stores and can easily stow away in the car boot. They also add greatly to the way of life in camp, remove backaches and provide a good surface on which to prepare meals. Clearly for the group camp a larger table and more chairs are necessary, but even if you do not take sufficient for one each, a basic system is better than nothing.

Even if you are able to light a fire and plan to cook some meals in true 'backwoods' spirit, it is still necessary to take a more convenient form of stove. The two main alternatives are the 'primus', using paraffin as fuel, and camping gas stoves such as calor or gaz. Personal preferences and availability are considerations although gas is probably simpler to use and highly reliable. Most camp sites stock gas and on the Continent 'Gaz' is certainly most popular. It has the big advantage of coming in several sizes of container, from the small backpacker's stove, with gas cartridge attached, to the larger cooking platform, with two or more burners and a rubber/plastic hose connecting to a cylinder of gas.

Cooking utensils are traditionally a 'nest' of billie cans or mess tins, similar to those issued to the Armed Forces. These can easily be loaned (Scouts, Services) but just as serviceable will be the household saucepans, kettle and stewpot. They do not pack quite so easily and take more room in the luggage; hence the preference for traditional gear.

What else should we take? This may depend on the camping site. Many official grounds have areas for personal washing, washing up and other functions for which equipment is needed if facilities are not present. Washing bowls, water containers for carrying and storage, a clothes line . . . think of everyday living and plan accordingly. Make a list of items for the camp and an additional list of personal items for each camper. Such a list might read:

Camp Equipment
Tents and Flysheets (complete)
Spare pegs, guylines & fastenings
Mallet
Water containers
Cooking stove and tools
Fuel
Food
Cooking pans & frying pan
Kettle
Catering aids – knives, fish slice,
  wooden spoon, etc.
Can/bottle opener
Scissors
Mirror
Washing-up liquid
Soap powder
Pot cleaners and dishcloth
Tea towels
Torch
Spare batteries
Camping gas light
Camping table
Camping chairs
Polythene bags – assorted
Clothes pegs
Clothes line
Trowel or small spade
Toilet paper
Needles and repair materials
Matches
Maps and compass
First aid kit
Whistle
Repair kit for airbeds

Personal Gear
Sleeping bag or blankets
Camping mat or air bed
Washing kit
Towels
Spare trousers, shirts,
  underwear, socks
Sleeping wear
Sweater and sweatshirt
Woollen hat and gloves
Handkerchieves
Swim wear
Plimsolls or track shoes
Wellingtons
Waterproofs
Anorak
Comb and nail brush
Cutlery, plate, bowl and
  cup
Penknife
Camera and films
Binoculars
Books and games
Notebook, pencil,
  coloured feltpens, art
  materials, drawing
  block
Sunglasses
Personal medications

Camp food

Hungry mouths need filling but camp food should be appetising, well cooked and varied. Porridge, beans, bread and jam can all be very pleasant and have their place on the menu but can become monotonous if presented every morning to the breakfasting camper. Where possible fresh food should be used, but under many camp situations this may not be possible for all meals. Tinned and other processed foods are fine but often bulky to carry and very heavy. Dehydrated foods are highly suitable for the lightweight camper but need to be treated with care in preparation. For general camp purposes you can often go to the local shops or camp store and purchase food as required. Meals are then similar to those at home and can be varied and form a balanced diet.

One should always try to eat a good breakfast which will give plenty of energy for hikes and camp activities for the day. A light lunch, either in camp or packed for travelling, is best, since heavy mid-day meals tend to produce afternoon slumber! A light tea can be taken on return to camp while awaiting the main evening meal, which is best eaten early (and particularly during daylight hours). A light supper can be arranged if needed before bedtime. In this respect hot drinks are good food value, can be filling and quick to prepare. They should also be varied.

A typical camp menu should also include some fibre (roughage) provided by fresh fruit (apples, oranges), dried fruit (prunes), green vegetables or bran-based cereals, since constipation in camp can easily occur. Most of these foods also provide essential vitamins.

If you have a permanent camp and weight is not a problem then fresh foods together with normal routine shopping will supply your needs. However, today there are specialist preparations of dehydrated foods, many of which supply the big expeditions. They are often costly and not so readily available, but it is possible to plan camps using dehydrates with normal shopping in mind. Some food that we often eat at home is of course dry or dehydrated already – packet soups, dehydrated potato and other vegetables, rice, spaghetti, pastas, packet meals (curries, Chinese, etc.), dried milk, packet puddings, and I can only suggest a walk around a large supermarket with an eye for convenient camp foods. It is possible to carry your own food supplies for several days if you plan your meals carefully in this way. The backpacker always has to consider weight before other factors in food and equipment and in planning a large scale expedition, food for several members over several weeks can be carried with you into relatively remote areas, where local food costs may be high and availability limited. Meals should still be as interesting and appetising as possible, although some individuals in the group may well consider dry packet foods do not look (or taste) as good as fresh meat and vegetables. It is advisable while preparing and cooking such meals carefully to read and follow any instructions provided on the packet. Some such foods can also be given an enhanced flavour by adding an Oxo or other meat extract, or curry powder if others find this tasty.

Everyone should be given a task in the camp meal – preparation, fires, cooking, washing up, clearing away – and nobody should be exempt. There will always be those who say, 'I haven't done it before', often with reference to washing up, and the boys may well feel the girls are better suited to many tasks. But young boys in wheelchairs can wash or dry cutlery and plates, and mentally retarded adults can empty food out of tins as well as you or I. There is no need for staff to do everything and it is very undesirable that we should even think this way. Camp life is for everyone and is one of the best sources of independence training that I know. The spirit to help and be involved is usually very strong and there is always a job for everyone. A camp rota of duties and tasks is therefore beneficial to all, but put group members in pairs where possible. The job gets done a lot quicker and everyone learns co-operation.

Cooking meals over a camping gas burner presents few problems but this is less true if you are planning to use a woodfire. The wood will need to be dry, both for lighting and burning, and some woods burn better than others. Softwoods, such as larch, pine or fir, burn fast and produce a lot of flame; they are suitable for starting a fire. Hazel, birch and twigs from hedgerows are also good kindling fuel but away from the forest you may have to be more adaptable and burn dried heather or gorse. Hardwoods such as beech, ash and oak are good once the fire has started and burn slowly for longer cooking times. A good bed of hot ash is needed before you can boil water and cook the meal and a support for pans will have to be made from large logs or stones. Wood smoke smells fine, especially from a distance, but does get in your eyes, making them smart and water, and makes food taste 'different'. A good wood source is necessary and must be collected before the fire is lit and the cooking begins. Camps at the coast can use driftwood fires and in forest situations you may find firewood. Don't forget permission to light a fire and all the hazards associated with an open fire. If in doubt, don't light one!

The camp site

If you plan to stay on a permanent site you will have no problems in selecting your site, but camping in more open, wild places may present you with the decision as to where to pitch tents. The most scenic sites might well not be best for camping. Try to avoid any area likely to be wet or prone to flooding – bottoms of valleys, edges of streams, heavy clay soils. Look at the plants growing there – tussocks of reeds always indicate wet soils. Find a piece of level ground, preferably raised, protected from wind (and rain) by a hedge or wall, and where the drainage appears good. Position your tent so that the entrance faces away from the prevailing wind direction and preferably towards an interesting view. In exposed moorland and coastal districts the sparse trees will usually lean away from the prevailing wind and give you a guide on tent positions.

On some upland sites the ground may be very stony so that you cannot push tent pegs deep enough. Under such circumstances you may need to anchor the tent down with rocks or stones. A similar line of stones around the edge of the flysheet can help prevent wind blowing underneath or rain driving onto the tent itself. Stones can be used to construct a windbreak for your fire or stove. Make sure they are removed from under the tent itself.

Look for your water supply, and if you plan to cook on an open fire check your source of fuel. Remember you have to get all your gear to the site, so if you plan to use a vehicle make sure it can get all the way there. Similarly, if your campers have mobility problems, think of the ground with respect to access for both wheelchairs and walkers.

Handicapped people can camp in wild country but planning needs to be more precise and all eventualities must be considered wherever possible. On arrival at the site first pitch the tents, so that in the event of rain you can put your other gear under cover immediately and keep dry yourselves. Do not unpack, lay out sleeping bags and clothes, or start the meal. Likewise, at the end of camp leave tents standing until the end; pack bags and rucksacks under cover of the tent. Always erect the fly sheet over the tent, leaving the correct space between the two layers. Waterproofing is provided from the flysheet – the tent by itself will leak, certainly at the seams. If it continues to rain and water accumulates under the tent groundsheet, consider digging a small ground trench at the rear and at both edges of the tent to drain away water. Leave turfs turned aside at the edge of the trench in order to replace them when you eventually strike camp.

There are so many small hints and ideas that help to make life under tents more pleasant and comfortable. It can be fun, but it can be misery too. Good planning and organisation, a lot of thought before you go and consideration of your camp site will all help keep it fun!

Backpacking

The backpacker is a highly versatile camper. Travelling light he can reach more inaccessible places than other campers and often many miles from civilisation. In this respect backpacking may not be appropriate for many handicapped people, although clearly there will be others who can consider it.

Much of what has been said in earlier sections of this and the previous chapter can apply to this adventurous activity which clearly can be moderated and adapted to suit the participants. Roads, lanes and tracks can be followed rather than exposed rugged terrain, enabling the walker to move over easier surfaces. Distances travelled can be shorter and camps sited in more accessible places. Heavier gear could even be taken along by vehicle in advance, while the hiker only carries more essential items, but perhaps this should not then be thought of as backpacking. But do we need to use heavy gear? Can we keep the weight down sufficiently to enable handicapped people to carry their own camp equipment?

Much depends on the rucksack in which you will carry everything. It is important that it fits correctly and comfortably, with the weight distributed on your back and not hanging from the shoulders. Most backpackers therefore use a frame pack, although there are so many models and designs that the choice becomes difficult. You may find cost is one determining factor, although size of pack and shape of frame must be considered. The length of frame should be the same as the distance between your highest prominent neckbone and the top of the hip bone. Most of the pack is carried as high as possible, and a waist strap (hip belt) helps move the weight load to the hips and away from the shoulders. A foam padding under the shoulder straps helps prevent any rubbing and numbness in the arms and makes for more comfortable carrying. When the hip belt is fitted properly it should be possible to put your thumbs under the shoulder straps with ease, showing little weight is being taken by the shoulders.

Remember you are carrying the rucksack as part of your load, so choose one that is of lightweight but strong construction. The pack is usually of heavy-duty nylon (check the stitching where straps join the pack) and the frame of a light alloy. Packing the rucksack is equally important and the weight should be evenly distributed, with items needed first or most frequently packed last, where they can easily be found. For instance, your hike tent can be carried in a roll at the top of the pack, often outside, and strapped across, the pack itself. Similarly, the sleeping bag, which is bulky and difficult to pack inside the rucksack, may be placed in a waterproof stuff sack and hung below the main pack. Polythene bags are an essential item, and both your tent and sleeping bag should be wrapped within a large plastic 'bin liner' for added protection from rain. Clothes, food and other gear can also be packed inside polythene bags within the pack, enabling things to be found more easily as well as giving them some extra waterproofing.

Backpacking gear
Weight is important if everything is being carried on your own back. Manageable loads vary considerably depending on the

stature, age and sex of the backpacker but on average should be about 10–14 kg (20–30 lb). Only carry essential items, select lightweight products and share the load between members of the group. Make a list of gear which you feel is necessary and weigh individual items on the bathroom scales. Calculate the total and then begin to think how you can reduce the load. Some containers may be heavy and not required; food items may be changed for others; but some of the weight may simply be a feature of the particular equipment in your possession. You can do little about this except bear the fact in mind when buying gear.

Much importance is attached to the weight of the heavier items – a few kilos saved on a tent make up for all the grams on smaller items. Unfortunately lightweight hike tents tend to be far more expensive than more conventional models and a well-known name on a nylon 'two-man hike lightweight' will cost around £100. It is possible to purchase lower-priced tents with similar specifications, but one may not then obtain the same degree of waterproofing and find that seams leak in heavy rain. Similarly, strength of materials and stitching at stress points can let you down under severe weather conditions such as gale-force winds and driving rain.

One well known tent is particularly suitable for use by handicapped hikers and backpackers, or in a more permanent camp situation. This is the Vango Force 10 (Mark II Featherweight) in which the nylon tent is supported by A-poles at the front, an upright at the rear and a ridge pole. The access is consequently very good since there is no single upright in the centre of the entrance. A side guy holds out the inner tent to give more room inside by means of a fastening between the tent and flysheet. When closed the flysheet gives front storage space, ideal for the rucksack and cooking utensils. The weight complete is little over 3 kg (6 lb) and on larger Vango models an extension piece can also be fitted.

You may be lucky enough to locate a good quality used tent for about half the price through the advertising columns of the two principal outdoor monthly magazines for hikers and ramblers, *Climber and Rambler* and *The Great Outdoors*. Look at a wide range of makes and models at one of the Camping Exhibitions or at a well-stocked outdoor shop. In the summer visit a few camp sites and look at the names on tents which appear to suit your own purpose. Take advice from owners where possible and don't make up your mind too quickly.

Most other items of gear needed by the backpacker can also be used in conventional camp situations, and a useful check-list is given below.

Rucksack	Soft shoes – plimsolls
Lightweight tent	Spare clothes – trousers,
Sleeping bag	shirt, underclothes, socks
Sleeping mat	Handkerchieves
Cooking stove (Gaz)	Sweater
Cooking utensils	Waterproofs (lightweight) –
Plate, mug, cutlery	cagoule and over-trousers
Dehydrated foods	Torch
Washing kit	Maps and compass
First aid kit	Penknife
Repair kit	Can/bottle opener
Notebook and pencil	

Depending on individual items, especially the tent, quantity of food carried, cooking items and clothing, the total weight of the full pack can be in the region of 12 kg (23 lb).

Finally, footwear is probably the most important single factor to consider, although everything that was said on this subject when we looked at hiking and rambling will apply equally well here. Wear thick woollen socks over your normal pair which should be regularly changed, since this will help to avoid blisters. Foot washing and powdering every night will also assist in this respect, but nothing will stop ill-fitting boots from causing problems. Choose your boots with care, spend time in treating them with waterproofing materials and your feet will benefit accordingly.

Expeditions

In my earlier book in this series, *Out of Doors with Handicapped People*, I concluded with a short account of an expedition which I organised in 1977 for six physically handicapped young people. The venue for our scientific recordings was Switzerland, amidst the high snowy peaks of the Bernese Alps. We were not rock-climbing or mountaineering, nor canoeing on the fast-flowing rivers, but nonetheless the adventure and excitement achieved by the students was a highlight of their lives – and has probably influenced their development since the event.

The results of the expedition were fully published in a report, which contained both the scientific findings and a series of personal accounts by each student member of the team. Adventure here was high mountains, avalanches, glaciers and wild places – but mostly it was being there and fully participating. Henry, one of the group confined to a wheelchair, was particularly impressed with being able to sit, in pouring rain, at over 3000 metres beneath the towering mass of the Eiger and looking across a great expanse of glacier ice to see walls of snow falling away from the mountain edge. The rumbling noise sounded as thunder and could be heard from miles away. His comment was that he had never imagined seeing the very things he had previously only read about in his geography textbook!

Everyone, including all those needing wheelchairs, was taken to the highest points available – the Jungfrau at 4300 metres and Birg on the other side of the valley, by either mountain railway (similar to that on Snowdon in North Wales) or cable car. The wheelchairs were pulled out onto the glacier ice, while the walking members of the group staggered across rock scree slopes and along narrow mountain paths – often, at Birg, in thick mist conditions.

While it might not be possible for many people to climb mountains, it is often possible to explore them in other ways, and once on high to follow well pathed routes or to make descents to lower altitudes. Expeditions do, however, require considerable planning, and this one was no exception. One needs to obtain as much information on the area as possible, and in this respect the Embassy and Tourist Boards can be most helpful.

Travel considerations are especially important if you intend to take wheelchairs. It is also ideal if someone can visit the region in advance to ascertain any problems which may arise and to see what will be possible for exploration, adventure and study. This was possible in our first venture to the Alps but has not been a necessary feature of subsequent expeditions organised.

After two smaller and perhaps slightly less ambitious expeditions, we decided in 1981, as part of the International Year of Disabled People, to celebrate with an exciting adventure in the Outer Hebrides, on the islands of Harris and Lewis. Once again the handicapped young explorers were selected from the same special school and were all bright and alert but limited in mobility. Although there were no wheelchair users it should be remembered that the person confined to a wheelchair will go anywhere that the able-bodied 'pusher' can take him, while the person with limited, staggering movement has to give all of the effort himself to traverse rough ground and climb mountains.

Planning again began early in the previous year and after meeting the students selected we were certain that once again the expedition would be a great success – an event in their lives. It is satisfying that of the six Alps adventurers five proceeded to studies at University and it can be argued that their experiences on the expedition helped them establish themselves in their new world.

Our selected base on the islands was an expedition hut used by other young people and very well furnished and located for outdoor studies. In the Alps we had decided to camp, and consequently far more gear had to be taken in the vehicles. Living in tents can be fun but organisation must be good if chaos is to be avoided, especially when one is trying to produce academic results in addition to creating a spirit of adventure. Certainly a hut enables workers to sort out their findings from the day's field work, use equipment such as a microscope, keep books and notes and find things again! There is a tendency in a tent for everything to disappear under the groundsheet! The working day also becomes extended when you have electric lights, although we did find Gaz lamps ideal for late night sessions when living in tents.

Projects on Harris centred around island history and geography, together with natural history studies on the marine life of the rocky shore and surveys of the plants, insects and birds of the sandy machair and the peat moorland. Remote coastlines and barren moorland are ideal scenes for adventure and memories, as Jackie found out when she fell into a peat bog, on the very first evening, complete with smart, white trousers! In their personal accounts, published in the final report, Phillip remarks that 'the going was often very rough and it proved a great challenge to us all. The highlight of this was when we went right to the top of a very steep hill while collecting insects. It took us a few hours and although I fell over on numerous occasions, often in boggy areas, I enjoyed it immensely'. For Phillip, that hill was his Alpine mountain and his challenge was that climb . . . under his own steam! It is interesting that he also felt the hut enabled him to enjoy the expedition more, and that, although he spent a night under canvas on the moors, two weeks like that might well have changed his feelings on the entire expedition.

We were also able to introduce them to island life. The ways of the crofter, the remoteness and simplicity of their existence, were quite new concepts to them all. Sitting each evening by the warmth and glow of a peat fire, without the influence of television, talking of how they might enjoy and cope with such a lifestyle, it became apparent that, while a short exposure may be thought of as fun, longer periods might well prove very different. Tracy realised that the whole way of life seemed rather rough and hard work, and that while she would have liked to live as a crofter for a short time, she was uncertain about it indefinitely. Phillip felt that he would 'miss a lot of things – English sport, television and the general everyday life I am used to'.

An expedition provides many outlets for the development of personality, social independence, inter-relationships and other social skills, within the framework of adventure and excitement. It has a role to play in the total development of the individual, a factor which is well appreciated within the Duke of Edinburgh Award Scheme. The expedition features at Bronze, Silver and Gold Award stages, with progressive levels of difficulty and achievement. Varying means of travel can be involved – hiking, cycling and canoeing are chosen as examples, but other outlets could also be considered. The distance which handicapped adventurers must cover will vary depending on the degree of disability, but the aim is that participants should complete the basic pattern of the scheme whenever possible. The Youth Service Officer of the Local Education Authority will be able to assist anyone interested and often someone may be responsible for organising the programme for handicapped young people.

The Award expedition requires considerable evidence of planning and consideration of travel, terrain, equipment and a topic for particular study 'en route'. Trial expeditions are undertaken before the attempt on the assessed final one is made. At the Gold stage this must be undertaken in 'wild country', a list of which is given in the Handbook. Much of what has been stated in other parts of this book will apply to many aspects of the Award scheme, but a special publication is available from their offices which has particular relevance to handicapped adventurers.

8   Reaching high and low

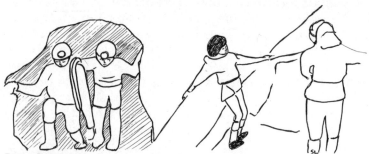

Introduction

Jane closed her eyes. The world stopped spinning beneath her feet. She took a deep breath, and tentatively opened her eyes again. The rough granite of the rock face was two inches from her nose. She slowly tilted her head and looked up, following with her eyes the rope attached to her waist belt up the rock to the large flat shelf a few feet above her. The nylon climbing rope stretched on upwards past the worn toe of a large boot, and disappeared from view. Five and a half feet beyond the boot Jane could see the face of the climbing instructor, grinning with encouragement. 'Are you coming up, lass, or d'you want to eat your lunch right there?'

'Don't rush me!' cried Jane. 'I'm trying, I'm trying!' She wriggled the fingers of her left hand into the horizontal crack in the rock. Nervously she let go her secure hold with her other hand and crawled her fingers slowly up the rock.

'Further!' called the instructor. Jane licked her lips and reluctantly stretched her hand higher.

'That's it, now right!' She inched her hand sideways. 'No, the other way.' That voice again! Her hand slid back across the uneven rock. 'That's it, you're there!'

'Not there,' denied Jane.

'Yes, it's only a small hold,' replied the instructor.

Jane pressed two fingers into a tiny indentation in the rock. Her elbow shook. She slowly dragged her right foot up the rock until she felt a shallow ledge beneath it. Transferring her weight, she dug her fingers tighter into the rock and pressed on her right leg. The left foot crept up the rock, and stopped. Jane risked a downward look. Her boot was two inches below the ledge, and only a foot below her left hand. Her right knee trembled in violent spasms. 'I can't do it!' she cried.

The reassuring voice of the instructor floated back. 'Oh yes you can, push with your right leg.' Jane tensed and pushed her right leg. The left boot miraculously slipped up the rock securely onto the ledge. She pulled her left hand from the rock and straightening up, thrust it high to grab the top of the rock face. With a shout of glee she threw her other hand to the top and, pressing hard on her hands, scrambled excitedly, and in a most undignified manner, up and over to sprawl in a sweating, panting heap at the feet of the imperturbable instructor.

'Well done!' he exclaimed.

'I did it! I DID IT!!' Jane screamed, and dragged herself to her feet by grabbing handfuls of the instructor's clothing. She hugged him tearfully and beamed up into his smiling face. 'Did I do it?' she demanded.

'You surely did!' came the understated reply, giving her a responsive hug with rope-entwined arms. The instructor felt as proud as Jane at her achievement, for Jane is a Down's Syndrome lady, living in a hospital ward for mentally retarded adults, whose most exciting moment in her 38 years had been paddling at the water's edge on her annual visit to the seaside. For Jane, this rock-climbing adventure had tested her courage more than anything in her life, and she was remarkably restrained in her expressions of elation, satisfaction and achievement.

This is not intended to be a treatise on how to climb rocks. There are already a number of excellent books (a selection is listed in the Appendix) which between them provide a comprehensive guide to rock climbing techniques. In any case for the novice climber no written work could ever replace learning by experience in company with more knowledgeable and experienced climbers. This chapter is therefore written with three different types of reader in mind: the experienced climber who wishes to supplement his knowledge to enable him to instruct with more confidence a group of novice handicapped climbers; people involved with handicapped children or adults who are not themselves climbers, but may wish to seek out a climber to introduce them to rock climbing; and the disabled person who would like to climb and can similarly give advice to his or her instructor.

For most people, rock climbing has an aura of danger about it. Their vision of rock climbing is coloured by books, television and newspaper accounts of daring expeditions assaulting hitherto unconquered peaks, by feats of courage, determination, endurance, strength and skill, usually necessitating vast quantities of equipment supplied by wealthy sponsors. Although one may ultimately aspire to such grandiose schemes, one need not begin quite so lavishly. It may be of comfort to know that the great British climber Joe Brown began climbing, according to his autobiography, using his mum's washing line as a climbing rope. However, although washing lines are definitely not recommended, rock climbing is an activity which can be undertaken in conditions of apparent danger and can provide a challenge to be overcome only by courage and determination. The attributes of endurance, strength and skill need not be present but can be acquired by most people if they have the desire and determination.

If conducted sensibly, with proper regard to safety, rock climbing for beginners need not be at all dangerous, and a physical handicap need not prevent a person rock climbing, or at least have the experience of moving up a rock face. Requirements are appropriate equipment, properly used; suitable staff; a location and climb suited to the abilities and disabilities of the handicapped students, and the aims to be met; and correct safety procedures to be observed at all times.

Climbing gear

For most climbs the handicapped person can wear the same clothing as for other outdoor activities such as hiking, rambling and backpacking (see chapter 6).

Climbing boots with good ankle support and rigid commando-pattern vibram rubber soles are suitable, but other hiking boots or gym shoes could be considered acceptable alternatives. It is important that the climber is warm enough and good wool clothing is as essential as when hiking in wild country. When waiting to climb there is little sustained physical movement to keep one warm and the principle of wearing several layers of clothing applies just as much as for other activities. A woollen hat can be worn but during the climb a proper helmet (BS.4423), correctly adjusted and secured, is essential for both instructor, assistant and climber.

Gloves may be worn for belaying or abseiling, but unless needed for medical reasons are often a hinderance when climbing. However, for extreme conditions fingerless mittens are a useful compromise. During belaying and classic abseils the friction of the rope burns nylon and PVC anoraks and cagoules and consequently a thick sweater or tough cotton anorak should be worn.

The equipment must be in good condition, inspected regularly and adequate for the climbs undertaken. This is especially true for the ropes which, although of nylon, do stretch considerably during a climb and become abraded against rock surfaces. The climbing rope must be changed regularly, depending on usage. Information on ropes can be obtained from the major equipment stores listed in *Climber and Rambler* each month.

Waist ties

a   *End of rope*: this traditional and simplest way of tying the end of the rope round the waist by means of a bowline, although safe and cheap, has disadvantages. The rope cannot be disconnected quickly; the climber cannot be transferred to another rope or belay quickly or easily; the narrow rope is uncomfortable when climbing, and painful in a fall.

b   *Waist length*: the narrow hemp line is wrapped around the waist five or six times, knotted with a reef knot, and the ends tucked in between the strands. The climbing rope can be tied on direct using a bowline or figure-of-eight, or via a karabiner.
Advantages: the line is cheap; easy to attach; easy to see from a distance if it is worn correctly; easy to check visually for wear and tear; and spreads the load around the waist.
Disadvantages: it should be replaced each year if used frequently; the knot is easy to untie (potentially a problem with maladjusted or some mentally handicapped students); once popular with outdoor education centres, the waist length has been largely superseded by the Swami belt or waist belt.

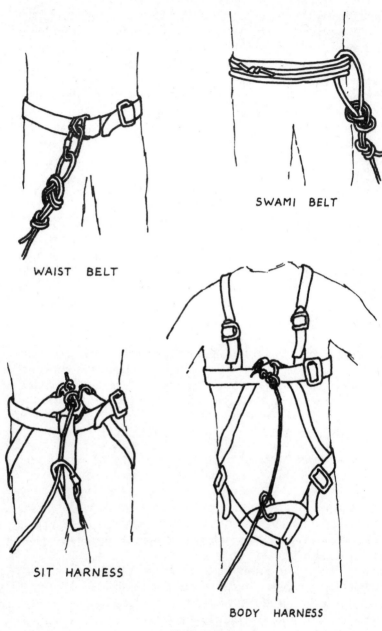

WAIST BELT

SWAMI BELT

SIT HARNESS

BODY HARNESS

Waist ties

c   *Swami belt*: a nylon tape is used around the waist similar to a hemp line.
Advantages: it is easy to check visually for wear and tear; and spreads the load around the waist.
Disadvantages: the ring bend or tape knot is awkward to tie tightly and correctly; if tied incorrectly, the tape will slide loose, and it is not easy to see from a distance if the knot is tied correctly.

d   *Waist belt*: usually two inch nylon webbing with a protective canvas sleeve fastened by a buckle. A movable 'D' ring enables the climbing rope to be attached (usually with a figure-of-eight) via a karabiner.
Advantages: the load is spread evenly around the waist; it is easy to see from a distance that the climbing rope is attached correctly; it is also easy to transfer to another rope.
Disadvantages: the canvas sleeve prevents examination of the webbing; the tail of the belt easily frays and makes fastening difficult; it is difficult to fasten tightly; if not fastened correctly the belt can come undone; in use the buckle is usually out of sight of the climb leader, thus preventing a visual check on the fastening; waist belts come in various lengths or 'sizes' and a selection may have to be provided.

Two disadvantages of all the above waist attachments are that there is no body support and the attachment is invariably pulled uncomfortably high in use. This is especially pronounced for rotund climbers!

e   *Sit harness*: this is of nylon webbing, rather like a waist belt with additional webbing around the thighs and up between the legs. The climbing rope is tied directly on through webbing loops with a bowline and threaded through a lower karabiner.
Advantages: easily checked visually for correct fastening and rope attachment; it need not be adjusted as tightly as the waist-only attachments; the harness does not pull up as far; it is more comfortable; although made in various sizes, each size is very flexible in use, and although comfort may suffer, safety is maintained.
Disadvantages: the straps between the legs can cause discomfort to men on a fall, especially if the harness is not the correct size –

this can be lessened by omitting the lower karabiner, without loss of safety; when there is a strong pull on the climbing rope, climbers who are very top-heavy or have poor back control or weak limbs may fall backwards away from the rock – this can be avoided for most people by omitting the lower karabiner; the thigh straps can hook onto rock projections; it is difficult to transfer to another rope; climbers with weak hips must have the waist part of the harness around their waist clear of their hip bones – with bulky clothing this can sometimes be very difficult and awkward; sit harnesses are more than twice the price of waist belts.

f   *Body harness*: a full harness of nylon webbing giving support around the thighs, back, chest and shoulders. The climbing rope is attached directly to the harness at the chest and threaded through a lower karabiner.

Advantages: for the climber – or indeed anyone – who 'enjoys being trussed up like an oven-ready chicken', this is a most stimulating experience; the device can be used as an emergency stretcher or as part of a stretcher; the body harness gives considerable support (both physical and moral) to climbers with weak limbs, or, like thalidomide young adults, missing two or more limbs and unable to use false limbs, or climbers with weak or distorted backs such as may occur with spina bifida; it also enables grossly handicapped people – usually youngsters – who have seen their less handicapped friends climbing and wish to emulate them and experience the same feelings of achievement and satisfaction, to be hauled bodily up the rock face. This may not be climbing, but it is certainly a wonderful experience.

Disadvantages: there are, strangely enough, many climbers who derive little enjoyment from being comprehensively trussed up, and find the harness too restrictive; even with practice, attaching the body harness is a long and arduous process (it is often easiest to lay out the harness on the ground, then lower the climber into the webbing); because of the vast number of straps and buckles, the fastenings need to be checked and double-checked. It may be both an advantage and a disadvantage that once on correctly, the body harness cannot be easily removed.

Belay techniques

a *Dynamic belay*: the live rope is passed around the belayer's body and turned round his forearm.

Advantages: the standard procedure for most climbers; no devices to hinder movement or to go wrong; a great deal of control for letting out and taking in; very sensitive – even if the climber cannot be seen, his movements can be felt on the rope; easy to disconnect.

Disadvantages: may cause rope-burn if long sleeves are not worn; will damage nylon or plastic anoraks by friction heat.

There is a recent trend towards the use of mechanical belaying devices ('auto belayers') which are all friction devices. The most popular is the Sticht Plate.

b *Sticht Plate*: this is a bar or round plate with a slot, through which a loop of the climbing rope is fed and clipped into a karabiner. The model with a spring is probably better as this prevents the plate from jamming against the karabiner. The karabiner may be attached to the belayer's harness or waist ties, or directly to belay points. The braking effect can be increased by using two karabiners, and/or by incorporating a body belay.

Advantages: less strain on the 'inactive' arm; useful for a light belayer belaying a heavy climber.

Disadvantages: movement of the rope through the device is quite slow unless the optimum angle is used – this angle is particularly difficult to maintain when belaying an abseil; when the sticht plate is connected to the waist, the body tends to be pulled into an uncomfortable stooped position; clothing and the securing cord can be dragged into the plate, reducing friction; the braking arm needs free movement beside and behind the body which is not always available; the device is awkward when used with hawser-laid ropes.

c *The Italian Hitch*: this is a simple friction knot around a pear shaped karabiner or a figure-of-eight descendeur, popular among continental climbers.

Advantages: very effective – a fall can be arrested with one hand.

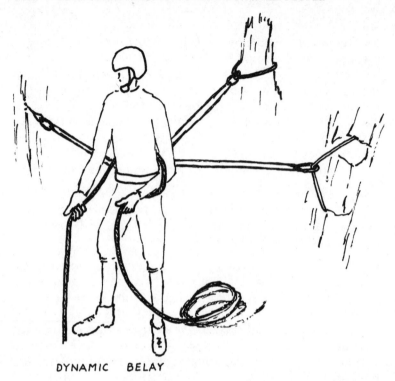

DYNAMIC   BELAY

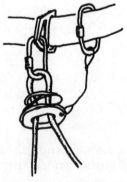

STICHT   PLATE

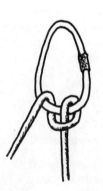

ITALIAN   HITCH

Belay techniques

Disadvantages: tension must be maintained on the 'live' rope to prevent the knot moving out of position – this is fine for belaying a smooth flowing rock 'tiger', but not for belaying a hesitant novice; it is not suitable for hawser-laid rope.

Climbing Helmets

It is surprising that there is much argument and controversy about whether or not helmets are desirable. The head is the most vulnerable part of the body and it makes sense to protect it accordingly. Serious injuries to the head can be, and all too frequently have been, caused by falling rocks and even small pebbles, by falls of only a few feet, by a climber swinging pendulum-like from a traverse, by slipping upside down on an abseil, or from dropped equipment. Whilst no helmet can provide absolute protection, it will absorb a lot of energy and thus prevent injury from most causes, and minimise injury from a severe blow.

The helmet should have these characteristics: comply with BS 4423; have an energy-absorbing lining; give all-round protection (crown, forehead, behind the ears, and down the back of the head as far as possible); allow good head movement and vision; have strong, comfortable fastenings (many climbers insist on a chin cup).

The most comfortable and secure helmets are those made for specific head sizes, but this provision is usually impractical when supplying helmets for a group of novices. There is a wide range of helmets available with adjustment for different size heads, but care must be taken to ensure a correct fit.

Descendeurs

These are friction devices used for abseiling or lowering.

a   *Figure of Eight Descendeurs*:
Advantages: the most fool-proof and safest of all the descendeurs; sufficient metal to dissipate heat; easy to assemble and operate; sufficient friction braking for a comfortable descent; can be locked by jamming the control rope across the top, or by tying off with a bight of rope in a half-hitch, or by wrapping the control rope around the thigh.

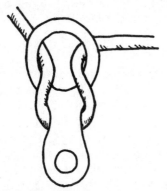

FIGURE OF EIGHT

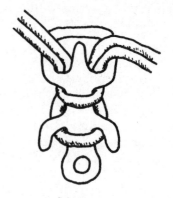

FAMMU

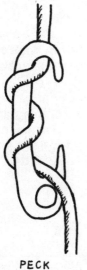

PECK

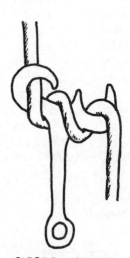

PIERRE ALLAIN

Descendeurs

b   *Fammu Descendeur*: operates on the same principle as the Figure of Eight, and when two abseil ropes are used it has the added advantage of separating them as they pass through, thus facilitating an easy pull.

c   *Peck Descendeur and Pierre Allain Descendeur*: both devices have a danger of the rope coming off if the load is released. Definitely not recommended for the inexperienced novice.

Disadvantages of all descendeurs: care is needed to prevent clothing from becoming pulled in and jamming the rope; many novices tend to hold the device with their free hand, thus jamming the rope with their fingers.

Knee and Ankle Pads
These provide useful protection for people who are susceptible to injury or need to use their knees a lot.

Staff
When undertaking rock climbing and associated activities with disabled people it is assumed that the activity will be led by at least two experienced climbers (although one of them may only be proficient at belaying), plus additional staff in appropriate numbers who can play useful and often invaluable supporting roles even if they themselves are not climbers.

There are many experienced climbers who climb to very high standards, but who find it difficult to adjust their techniques and attitudes when instructing handicapped novices. A suitable instructor would be experienced in climbing and improvised rescue techniques; safety conscious; flexible in his other approach; able to select climbs of suitable standard; very patient; and would know his or her own limitations and not be tempted to exceed them while in charge of the students.

Contact with suitable climbers may be made through outdoor education centres, colleges of education which run courses in outdoor education, county youth organisers, county outdoor pursuits organisers and the British Mountaineering Council. Other possible sources include climbing clubs, climbing magazines and climbing equipment shops, but climbers met in this way may not necessarily be suitable. Sheffield Adult Training Centres have an active outdoor pursuits scheme with a strong element of rock climbing.

Climbing skills

The activity of rock climbing can be used as a recreational activity for its own sake, as one aspect of a multi-discipline course or programme, as an exercise in assessment, or as a tool for training specific or general skills.

Many staff of Adult Training Centres for mentally retarded adults have found that rock climbing develops self-confidence and manipulative skills of trainees, and, most significantly, that these attainments during climbing are maintained and transferred to the work and social aspects of their centre.

Self confidence can be gained by achievement; not just by overcoming fear to reach the top of a climb, but also by making the dozens of small moves needed to accomplish the whole climb. The key to ensuring satisfaction and increasing confidence is to make the climb, however short, be within the means of the climber, or conversely to make the climber, if necessary with help, capable of completing the climb.

Manipulative skills, body awareness, co-ordination and balance are all crucial to climbing, and climbs can be selected to provide practice in specific skills.

Handholds: flat hold (pressing with the hand or fingers and pulling with the arm), finger hold (as for flat holds and in addition utilising limited parts of the finger or fingers), incut hold (grasping and pulling), pressure hold (pressing, often developing from a flat hold), mantleshelf (co-ordinating in sequence pulling and pushing actions of the whole body), pinch grip (opposed pressure of fingers/thumb or fingers/palm), undercut hold (pulling), side pull (sideways or horizontal pull), layback (sustained co-ordination of side pull with the arms and pushing with the legs), finger-, hand-, fist- and arm- jamming (finger and wrist and arm control, muscle strength), hand traversing (virtually reliant on hand and arm control and strength), wriggling, backing and bridging (total body control and co-ordination using opposition pressure in combination with other holds).

Most of the handholds described can also be used as footholds using much the same means of control but with feet and legs. There is no reason why someone whose leg, feet and toes are more manipulative than his arms and hands shouldn't climb bare-foot.

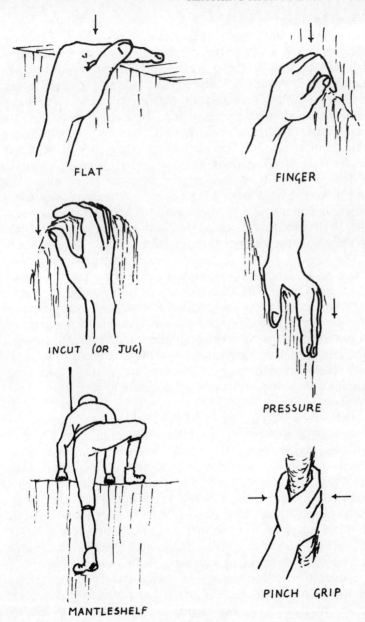

FLAT

FINGER

INCUT (OR JUG)

PRESSURE

MANTLESHELF

PINCH GRIP

Handholds (1)

Where to climb

The climbing area needs to be selected with care. Access is important. It must be borne in mind that many disabled people will find the walk to the crag far more difficult than the climb itself. Rough ground can literally be a stumbling block. Stiles may be a new and traumatic (or exciting) experience for many over-protected handicapped people. Your climbing group may well include children and adults who have been so protected by well-meaning parents or institutions that they have never before walked along anything more uneven than a pavement, and may need lots of encouragement to overcome their fear and lack of confidence. Wheelchairs, particularly with over-weight occupants, are very awkward to carry long distances. It may be decided that reaching the climb is to be an integral part of the whole rock climbing experience, and is treated as such.

For novices it is usually best to choose a crag or quarry with single-pitch climbs (10–15 metres) utilising a top rope with good belay points. Ideally there would be a number of climbs within a small area, and sufficient staff and equipment to provide several climbs (and associated activities) operating simultaneously, each with a minimum of two experienced climbers in charge. This would avoid the problem of what to do with those members of the group not actually climbing. Alternatives worth considering are climbing walls and sturdy trees.

The climbs need to be carefully chosen. The standard graded system is a useful guide – easy, moderate, difficult, very difficult, severe, very severe, hard very severe, and extremely severe. Generally for novices, climbs harder than easy, moderate and difficult are too challenging, and for some disabled novices, even the 'easy' grade climb may be beyond their capabilities; non-graded routes which experienced climbers may regard as scrambles could prove very suitable. Knowing the abilities and disabilities of the individual novice is most helpful in selecting a suitable route.

Difficulties of this nature can often be overcome by using a climb which has a variety of alternative holds or variations of route, and by using an experienced instructor to climb with the student, assisting to a greater or lesser degree. The instructor must use his own judgement to find the fine balance between

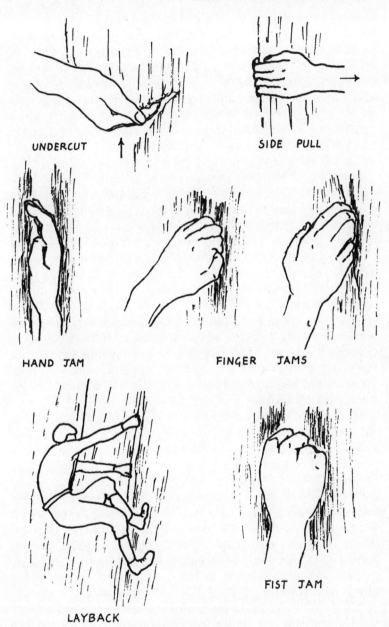

UNDERCUT

SIDE PULL

HAND JAM

FINGER JAMS

LAYBACK

FIST JAM

Handholds (2)

helping too much or too little – this is often the most crucial factor for the novice, determining whether he will be left with an impression of a tremendous adventure and with feelings of achievement, immense pride and satisfaction, or whether, at the other extreme, he will have feelings of deflation and anticlimax, or a traumatic experience of psychological mis-adventure. Verbal encouragement given quietly at close quarters rather than shouting from afar when the whole group can hear, is often the most effective assistance the instructor can give, particularly to mentally retarded climbers.

If the instructor does climb with the student, he must have provision to secure himself, either all the time or when appropriate. This could be in the form of a safety rope, chocks or slings, for example. He must be aware of the angle of the novice's top-rope, and avoid being knocked off balance by a pendulum swing when not himself secured. The instructor has a duty to himself, but more importantly to the group, not to be injured, and should not allow himself the luxury of taking risks. Especially for top-roping novices the belay should be very secure, using a minimum of two belay points. Three or more spread the load and reduce the risk of the belayer being pulled off balance. Efficient gloves are recommended. The instructor's safety rope should be attached separately. Equip-ment should be checked before and after use, particularly for abrasion and knots.

Most disabled novices climb very slowly, and the timetable will need to allow for this. An experienced climber's reactions and views of common sense will not necessarily be shared by a novice, and verbal reminders may not be enough. For instance the shout 'Below!' is often meaningless, and the instructor may well need physically to push a novice's head down and put his own arm across his neck for protection, as well as remembering to protect himself. Similarly, as one member of staff from an Adult Training Centre explained of a trainee: 'She has not yet formulised the cognitive concepts of left and right.' And as the trainee was also illiterate, writing 'R' and 'L' on her hands didn't help either!

Although desirable to introduce standard calls and correct technique (heels low, hands low, body away from rock, small steps, 3-point hold, planning ahead) at an early stage, it is by no

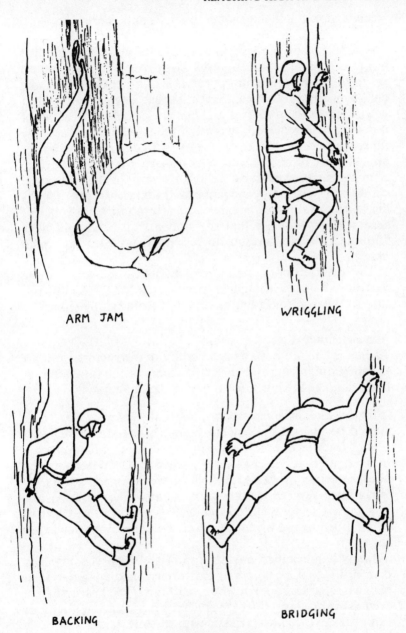

ARM JAM

WRIGGLING

BACKING

BRIDGING

Handholds (3)

means essential and may not be practical until more experience is gained.

After the climb (and when the cheers and applause have died away) ensure the student is well away from the edge and on easy ground before he unropes. This is potentially the most dangerous part of the climb: the student is usually still filled with euphoria and relaxes and becomes careless. Even when the waist tie is removed, the feel of the rope remains for some time, and in the excitement it is easy to forget you are no longer attached to a rope. The walk back down to the foot of the crag, even if on an easy path, can be more hazardous than the actual climb, so it is strongly recommended that the student retains his helmet and is accompanied by a responsible member of staff keeping so close that the student can be caught if he stumbles. Some circumstances may warrant a roped descent.

The members of the party not actually climbing, if near the foot of the climb, should keep well clear of the line of fire (not so much from falling bodies, but from falling stones!)

Associated activities

These are limited only by availability of instructors, suitable terrain, equipment, and the creativeness of the instructor. A few examples are given to stimulate the imagination.

Abseiling or Rappeling: a controlled slide down a rope. There should be at least one anchor point separate from the belay points for the double or single abseil rope. For novices a belayed safety rope, separately attached to the body, should be used. Students in wheelchairs can lower themselves on even fairly steep slopes, possibly with the assistance of a 'barrow boy' at first, as for stretcher lowering. The student will need to be strapped to the wheelchair, and the chair also attached to the safety rope.

Many handicapped novices appreciate the psychologically comforting presence of an instructor accompanying them (on his own separate rope) down the cliff face. The instructor can even assist by controlling the student's rope. Various methods can be used: the classic; classic with sit sling, harness or thigh loop; the sticht plate can be used as a descendeur, but probably

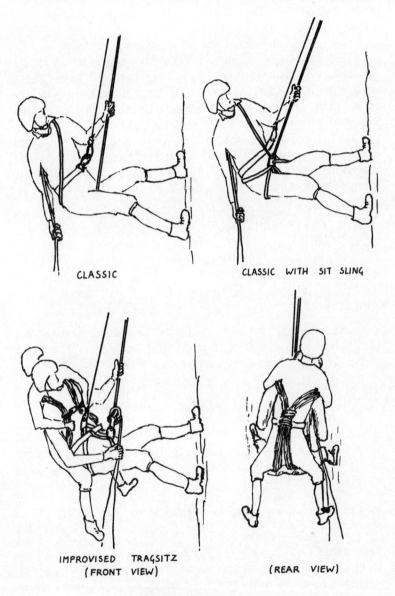

CLASSIC

CLASSIC WITH SIT SLING

IMPROVISED TRAGSITZ
(FRONT VIEW)

(REAR VIEW)

Abseiling techniques

the most suitable for novices is the figure-of-eight descendeur. The most comfortable attachment method is normally a sit harness or body harness.

Those who experience most psychological difficulty in commencing an abseil are a high proportion of mentally retarded novices. If it is decided to insist on the student experiencing this activity despite his opposition (and there are valid educational reasons for doing so) a number of variations are available. The student could commence from a sitting position, and perhaps use his feet later down the abseil when confidence grows. He could be held from behind by the instructor. The lower could be controlled from above. The instructor could carry the student in a tragsitz.

Improvised rescue techniques: prusiking (self-hoisting), using a variety of knots and devices. Assisted hoisting, using pulley hoist or stirrup hoist with assistance from above.

Lowering using karabiner brakes for example, operated from above. Stretchers and carries, using, for example, split rope carry, two man sling and pole carry, Pigott rope stretcher, Alpine basket.

Artificial climbing: probably not appropriate for novices, but very good exercises for developing self-reliance. Trees can prove suitable objects to climb in this way.

Aerial slide or ropeway: if it is to be really safe, galvanised aircraft wire ought to be used for the main structure. This is expensive but worth considering for a permanent structure. A less safe structure could still be used where a failure of the slide would not be dangerous, for example, over water (consider using life-jackets and/or rescue craft) or close to the ground parallel to a soft grassy slope.

Practice belay: use weights – bodies are more difficult to replace.

Traversing and boulder problems: excellent for practising technique. Firm discipline and a high staff:student ratio, ideally 1:1, is required. There is almost an inevitability about students gravitating upwards on a traverse, and this needs to be guarded against. A rope 'leash' could be used to physically prevent the student from climbing too high. In any case the instructor (or another student) should position himself below the climber to break his fall if necessary. Unroped traversing should not take place more than about four feet above the ground.

Gorge Scrambling: a combination of climbing and traversing along the rocky banks of a stream, trying, usually unsuccessfully, to avoid getting wet. Safety ropes may or may not be needed, but climbing or canoeing helmets ought to be worn. If ropes are needed, then their use is facilitated by all members of the party wearing waist-belts or harnesses throughout the activity.

River running: bouncing downstream with the current. Feet-first is the safest approach. Helmets and lifejackets must be considered essential, and wet suits highly desirable. If safety ropes are used, then care must be taken to ensure they do not become a hazard.

River crossing: various techniques can be practised, but the use of ropes on a suitable river can add to the illusion of danger while in fact minimising the hazards.

Scrambling: a scramble over rough terrain. This can be more dangerous than any of the above activities, and should be undertaken with great care. The staff must be continually vigilant and position themselves at all times to prevent or break a fall. Many disabled people have led very protected lives, and most have had little if any experience of walking over rough terrain. But with regular participation in scrambling, it is surprising how quickly confidence can be gained. A lot of individuals within institutional groups of mentally handicapped people almost automatically begin helping the less able members of the party.

Walking with ropes: each member of the party is tied onto one rope at intervals of about four metres (twelve feet), before commencing the walk or scramble. Best use of staff is made if they move independently and are free to assist where and when required. What is normally a fairly easy walk or scramble can be instantly changed into a difficult adventure. Woodland, small streams and bridges, stiles and narrow footpaths provide ideal obstacles needing thoughtful teamwork to negotiate. Most locations have variations of route to make the exercise harder or easier. The activity can be dangerous, for a slip by one student may pull all the other students off-balance, or a falling student may be held, but turned upside down in the process. Some students find this activity very frustrating, but when approached in the right frame of mind, it develops a team spirit very quickly and successfully.

Snow and ice climbing: ice climbing may not be suitable for handicapped novices, because of the relative inaccessibility of routes, the limited holds available on the route, and the dexterity required.

Snow climbing for students with good limb control is an activity worth considering, but as an exercise for its own sake, it can be boring for the novice.

Ice axe braking: a good safe run-off slope is essential. Without strong arm control, the ice axe would become a dangerous weapon, and tobogganing would be a much safer alternative. If you don't have a toboggan try using nylon anorak and over-trousers, or a bivvy bag!

Each activity can be complete in itself, or used in conjunction with others. The activities can be used as part of a larger exercise, be it an extended expedition on a grand scale, or simply a means of reaching an over-night stop in a tent, bivouac, igloo or mountain hut. Rock climbing and associated activities can be used as vehicles for self-improvement, as part of an assessment programme, or they can be undertaken purely for personal enjoyment. All the ingredients for achievement, satisfaction and fulfilment are there, and whatever the initial motive, it is rare indeed for anyone to complete their first climb and feel disappointed.

Caving
There is something compelling about cave exploration which evokes strong emotional sensations. The maze of dark underground passages made more menacing by deep flickering shadows from the lamp-light now illuminating, now con-

cealing, accentuating the mysteries of this other world. Fascinating rock sculptures intricately carved by underground rivers. The startling beauty of carbonate stalactites and stalagmites, siliceous fossils, cave pearls and other chemical and mineral formations. Puddles of water on the cave floor are often approached tentatively, with a suppressed fear of dropping into a bottomless pool. Sumps require an act of faith to duck into, never quite sure of resurfacing on the far side of the rock curtain. A narrow passage, and especially tight 'corkscrew' sections, are rarely entered without some doubt about whether the tunnel convolutions will prove too narrow for a safe return. For most people, caving is a thrilling experience containing a strong feeling of venturing into the unknown and of pitting your wits against the elements.

Caving and potholing are activities admirably suited to inclusion in a programme of adventure education. All the ingredients for excitement are there, and it must be one of the most immediate and compelling situations for teaching field studies. In addition, all members of the party are involved all of the time.

The suitability of these activities for people with handicaps is dependent on the type and degree of handicap and the nature of the cave. Few caves are suitable for transporting wheelchairs, but if the wheelchair user is able to crawl or drag himself along then he need not be excluded. Epileptics who recover within a short time are in no greater danger in most cave systems than they would be when hillwalking or rock scrambling.

Maladjusted children or others prone to hysterical fits can put themselves at risk, particularly if they have a tendency to attack other people or run off. I recall one memorable incident ten years ago when one small 13 year-old boy in a group of maladjusted lads, in the depths of a disused slate mine in North Wales, took an unreasoned and unprovoked dislike to another member of the party. It took four instructors to forcibly restrain him and tie him into a sleeping bag with a climbing rope. Even after carrying him to the surface, it was another three hours before he calmed down sufficiently to be released. Such a method of restraint may be necessary because of the difficulty of rescue underground.

Mentally retarded people have no physical difficulty with

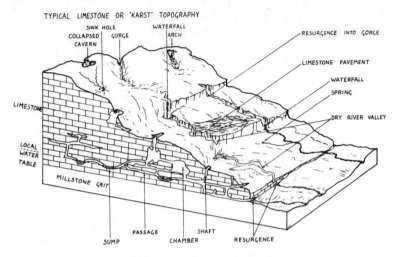

TYPICAL LIMESTONE OR "KARST" TOPOGRAPHY

Limestone cave landscape

caving except perhaps large size, and most get a huge amount of excitement and enjoyment from it. Any problems are usually of a psychological nature, and can nearly always be avoided or overcome by a high ratio of sympathetic staff. We must always remember that some people, handicapped or not, will find cave exploration to be claustrophobic and therefore frightening. In such circumstances the party should return to the surface, and I stress the need for a gentle approach. One reassuring measure is to link every member of the party to a length of rope and have experienced cavers or staff at regular intervals between the other participants. Many blind people enjoy caving in the company of sighted companions.

One experienced caver to each party may be sufficient in small cave systems but naturally the safety and flexibility is increased if more experienced cavers are present. It is recommended that at least two adults accompany a party of children. When leading a party of novices it is wise to enter only those caves with which you are familiar, or to enlist the help of guides from local caving clubs. These can be contacted through the National Caving Association. Caving parties should have at least four people, with a maximum of ten. Big groups should split up into smaller parties, each with their own experienced leader.

Suitable clothing and equipment is essential. The basic personal equipment for each caver should include warm clothes under a protective boiler suit, which may be bought from Services stores and similar local shops. Wet suits are highly desirable if immersion is anticipated. Boots are essential but different types are preferred for different situations – climbing ladders, negotiating narrow passages, climbing, wading. A useful compromise would have vibram soles with leather uppers and a metal toe-cap, but need to be tough. Hook fastenings for the laces should be avoided as the hooks often get caught on the side wires of lightweight ladders. A protective helmet is essential, with a chin strap and lamp bracket and an efficient headlamp. The lamp is usually carbide, or electric using a rechargable wet-cell battery. Dry cell batteries can be used, but they are generally less robust and have a shorter cell life.

Boiler suits can be improved to individual taste by elastic round ankles and wrists, straps under the feet, inside pockets under the arms, waterproof patches on shoulders and seat, and knee pads and elbow pads. Pads would probably be essential for non-ambulant cavers who do a lot of crawling. They can be of any suitable material such as neoprene or foam rubber, protected by leather, and may be sewn in or attached separately with straps. Gloves are useful when surveying or taking photographs, in order to keep the hands clean and help prevent mud getting onto the notebooks or camera.

Group equipment would vary according to the nature of the cave and whether potholing, vertical descent or ascent, is included. Most equipment is the same as that used for rock-climbing, with the possible addition of wire ladders, maypoles (scaling poles carrying a wire ladder), inflatable boats, or buoyancy aids. Diving equipment is often used, but this requires proper training and additional specialised equipment.

Emergency equipment should always be carried. This would include as a minimum: whistle, compass, notebook, pencils, first aid kit, carbide lamp, carbide, repair kit and spares for lamps, foods, can of fruit juice, bivvy bag. Suitable containers are canvas shoulder bags or waterproof army surplus ammunition cans.

Spelaeology, the study of caves, and biospelaeology, the

study of creatures that live in caves, are fascinating subjects in which most people can generate at least a passing interest. In caves, the effects of chemicals and minerals give rise to striking formations and the effects of water erosion are seen and felt in spectacular ways. Higher plants depending for life on photosynthesis are only found in the entrances to caves, but many lower plants (bacteria, algae and fungi) – the subterranean microflora – are found living in darkness.

The animal population of caves is quite varied. There are occasional visitors who enter accidentally, like certain flies, and live on the rich substrate at the cave mouth. Cave-dwellers by choice also exist outside, but thrive better living underground. These include bats and the insects which live on their droppings or guano. Some animals are genuine cave-dwellers, and live and reproduce underground. Terrestrial forms include earthworms, cave snails, insects, harvestmen and spiders. Aquatic cave-dwellers include several crustaceans, cave fish, and amphibians, although not all groups are represented in Britain.

Underground photography is a specialised activity of interest to many people. Hydrological measurement and recording, cave climatology, archaeology and surveying are all activities which can be enjoyed. A caving expedition could also include an overnight camp or bivouac underground to extend the experience.

Before embarking on any cave expedition, however short, at least one responsible person should be told the time of the party's departure; the precise location of the cave; and the estimated time of return. A wide time margin should be allowed, for progress is often very slow and tiring, needing frequent rests, and a minor accident such as a sprained or broken ankle may not need outside help but may delay the party considerably. Rescue operations involve a lot of people and should not be summoned unnecessarily. If the cave is liable to flooding then notice must be taken of recent weather and weather forecasts.

The major caving areas in Britain are in the limestone regions of South Wales, Northern Pennines, Derbyshire and Mendip Hills, with minor areas in North Wales, the Forest of Dean, Sutherland in Scotland and Furness in Southern

CLASSIFICATION OF BATS

Nasal membrane						RHINOLOPHUS (HORSESHOE)
No nasal membrane						
Tail goes outside the wing membrane			Tail completely enclosed within the uropatagium			
Half the tail outside interfemoral membrane	Tail outside interfemoral membrane 2 or 3 vertebrae		Ears joined at their base by a membranous band		Ears free	
	Wingspan 11 ins.	Wingspan 10 - 13 ins.	Ears also longer than forearm	Ears almost straight: dark colour	Tragus short and rounded at end: Wingspan 7-9 ins.	Tragus long and slender
TADARIDA	VESPER TILIO	EPTESICUS	PLECOTUS (Long-Eared)	BARBASTELLA	PIPISTRELLUS	MYOTIS (Natterer's, Daubenton's, and Whiskered)
					Wingspan 11 ins. Crown of head swollen MINIOPTERUS	
					Wingspan 11 - 16 ins. NYCTALUS	

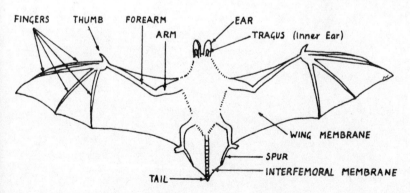

An identification guide to cave bats

Cumbria. There are also disused mines, notably in the Lake District, North Wales and Cornwall, but besides lacking the geomorphological interest, most have restricted access and all should be treated with considerable care and respect. Details of unfamiliar caves can be obtained from local clubs and in many cases caving handbooks.

There are show caves in most caving areas which are open to the public as tourist attractions and details can be found from local Information Centres. For severely handicapped people access to these is usually much easier and will give a great experience. Such caves do not require any special clothing or equipment and so may well be used to advantage to try out caving as an activity before investing in equipment; as a stepping stone to more adventurous caving; or for field study projects. Many caving areas also have dry river valleys and gorges formed by the erosion of the former cave roof. These, together with sea caves and large cave entrances, are often comparatively easier to approach and can be used in the same way as show caves.

9   Winter sports

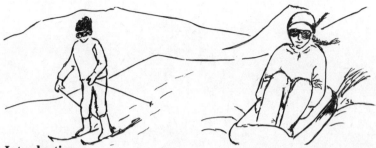

Introduction

The words 'winter sports' conjure up a vision of athletic people flying gracefully over ice or snow. Most people would therefore wonder how on earth a handicapped person could participate in sports such as skiing which require a high degree of co-ordination. The answer is that many handicapped people (and some quite severely so) can, and do, enjoy winter sports. Someone who has not experienced it cannot imagine the magic of gliding over snow, and the feeling of being on top of the world which comes with being high on a mountain in winter. As one young skier with cerebral palsy described it, 'All my life I've been trying to keep up with people, but when you are on skis you can go as fast.'

The benefits of winter sports for disabled people are not only those of a marvellous holiday in the fresh air, with all the new experiences of a winter resort, but there are immense physical benefits as well. It has been found that frequently people with conditions such as cerebral palsy are able to walk better after a skiing holiday and their co-ordination is often improved. To quote another young disabled skier, 'People look at it, you can do something the same as everybody else, and think – well – that must be quite something to actually ski.'

Keeping warm

Suitable clothing is very important for all outdoor activities and especially so for winter sports, particularly for a disabled person who may become chilled more quickly than an able bodied person who can move around more easily to keep warm.

It is not necessary to buy a large amount of expensive

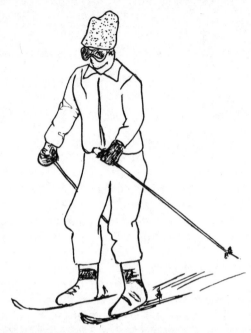

Warm clothing is essential for skiing

clothing, but the basic trousers and top must be good quality and waterproof, as conditions may be very wet and cold. Many sports shops will hire winter sports clothing, which may be a good idea at first. However, once the handicapped person has been bitten with the winter sports 'bug' it will probably be well worth buying an outfit. It is not necessary to buy from the pricey sports shops as several of the large chain stores now stock ski clothes. The important thing is to buy clothes designed actually for participating in winter sports and not ones which are made just to look good.

The essential items are as follows. A good windproof anorak is a must but can be attractive and be worn at other times. This must have a good zip and elasticated cuffs (which are often inner cuffs). This stops the snow from going up one's arms and is therefore very important!

Under the anorak it is better to wear two layers of thin jumpers than a thick one, so that one can be taken off if the weather becomes warmer. A thin polo-necked jumper or cotton shirt is useful as it helps to keep wind and snow out of one's neck.

Warm underwear is a good idea but it is important to find out what sort of temperatures will be expected; these can vary greatly with the area and time of year. Many layers of clothes would be needed in Scotland in January, but it might be very warm on the Continent in March.

A pair of waterproof trousers or salopettes (which are ski dungarees and are often padded,) are also needed. Salopettes are extremely warm and comfortable to wear and are very useful for sitting in a wheelchair out of doors on a cold day when at home!

Mitts or gloves which are waterproof will also be needed. Mitts are warmer than gloves, but are very clumsy and a handicapped person may find that he has difficulty in manipulations such as holding a ski stick whilst wearing mitts, so it is wise to try both. Also it is best to have ones which fit properly, as tight gloves make the hands colder, and mitts which are too large are very awkward. The mitts or gloves should be waterproof as they may spend quite a bit of time in the snow! Like the jacket sleeves they should have an elasticated cuff to prevent snow getting in them.

A woolly hat will be needed as it may snow heavily, or unfortunately even rain. Good sun glasses or preferably ski goggles are also required as the glare of sun and snow can be very painful and damaging to the eyes. Also important is a good sun cream (preferably one for higher altitudes) as the height and the glare from the snow can cause sunburn.

The other major item of clothing is suitable footwear. The warmest combination is two pairs of socks, one thin pair with a thicker pair on top. The type of boots worn will depend on the sports. Ski boots are needed for skiing and ski bobbing but a warm, lightweight boot such as a 'moon boot' will be useful for some activities or for wearing around the resort for shopping and so on. The latter are very good as they are warm, waterproof, comfortable and have a sole with a good grip. They are, however, not essential and other shoes with suitable soles can be worn, including wellington boots, with adequate socks to keep the feet warm, as wellingtons can be very cold.

As mentioned, a good pair of ski boots is essential for skiing or ski bobbing. These can be hired from ski shops or borrowed by holidaymakers with the Uphill Ski Club. (This Club for disabled skiers will be mentioned again later.) It is vital that ski boots fit very well, which may be difficult if the feet are an odd size or shape. Modern ski boots are quite high and very rigid. These may not be suitable for some types of disability because they are so hard and difficult to put on. The older type of leather boot may then need to be used, but these are not easy to obtain. However, most people will probably be able to manage a modern boot perhaps using some orthopaedic felt as padding. It is important to examine the feet every day to make sure that the boots are not chafing. This is vital if the feet are at all lacking in sensation, and great care must be taken to fit the boots carefully and not have any wrinkles in socks, as these can easily cause a sore.

Skiing
Skiing is a marvellous sport which can be enjoyed by people with many types of disability, for example the visually handicapped, mentally handicapped, those with some motor impairment such as cerebral palsy, the deaf, amputees and others. One young skier summed it up: 'I fell a lot but when I managed to go from the top of the slope to the bottom without a fault I felt I had really achieved something.'

People with different disabilities will need slightly different aids and anyone going skiing would be well advised to seek the advice of an expert.

The Uphill Ski Club has been taking disabled people on a skiing holiday on the Continent for seven years. Originally the Club was aimed at young people with cerebral palsy. However, it is growing rapidly and aims to provide recreational skiing for handicapped people with a variety of disabilities. The Club has a great store of experience gathered over the years, and has a range of different types of adapted equipment to help people with different needs. The Uphill Ski Club takes its own instructors on its holidays, and some of them have been coming as volunteers for several years so are very knowledgeable about teaching disabled people to ski. It also has a doctor, a nurse and a physiotherapist with each party.

The British Ski Club for the Disabled was founded in 1974

and has a great deal of experience with blind skiers and amputees. The Club also helps to train disabled skiers for competitive events such as the Winter Olympics for the Disabled, the first of which was held in Sweden in 1976.

Skiing in Britain can unfortunately be very cold. There are some very good areas in Scotland which have been developed as ski resorts. The largest of these is the Cairngorm area with Aviemore as the main resort. The weather in Scotland is very unpredictable and as mentioned, it can be bitterly cold. For this reason, sadly, it is probably not well suited for a disabled person to learn to ski, as initially quite a bit of time may be spent standing still or sitting in the snow! A continental resort towards the end of the season, when the sun should be quite hot, is ideal, as sitting in the snow can then be quite pleasant!

The other skiing available in this country is on artificial slopes. There are quite a few of these now throughout the country. However, they are really a poor substitute for snow, as they are very hard to fall on, which could put someone who is dubious about skiing completely off the idea. Snow, on the other hand, is soft and pleasant to fall on. The other main disadvantage of artificial slopes is that the method of getting back up the slope may not be suitable for many disabled people. Rope tows on matting are difficult to use and some slopes have nothing provided, it is left to the energetic individual to climb back up. This is a serious disadvantage to the more severely handicapped. However, the British Ski Club for the Disabled use artificial slopes quite extensively and for the blind and the physically handicapped with only a slight disability, or for amputees, they can be useful, especially for training for competitions.

Skiing on the Continent, as well as being warm, has the added excitement of a holiday abroad. Ski resorts are usually well supplied with other activities for evening entertainment, both for the energetic – swimming, bowling and discos – and for those who are too exhausted to do more than sit and have a drink. Austrian resorts particularly are well known for their delicious cakes, usually eaten with a cup of hot chocolate topped with a mountain of cream. This is most tempting after a day's skiing, and the mountain air seems to sharpen the appetite!

Before going on a skiing holiday it is a very good idea to do some pre-ski exercises regularly for some time before the holiday. Skiing uses muscles which may not normally be used and exercising will help to minimise pain and stiffness on the actual holiday. Pre-ski exercises for able bodied skiers can often be used, or advice may be sought from a physiotherapist for suitable exercises.

Ski Equipment

The equipment needed for a skiing holiday will vary with the individual handicap. The skis used may be of normal or near normal length for someone who is blind, deaf or slightly mentally or physically handicapped. These groups may also be able to use normal ski sticks. People with handicaps such as spasticity, may be much better using very short skis. These are much easier to turn for someone with not much strength in his legs. It has been found that it is often very helpful to tie the tips of the skis fairly closely together. This is done by drilling a hole in each ski tip and wiring them or tying them with a very strong cord. This is very useful if one leg is very weak as it keeps the weaker leg fairly near the stronger, but it does mean the skier will have trouble manoeuvring at places such the bottom of a ski tow. However, it would probably only be useful for people who have trouble manipulating their skis in these circumstances anyway. It can be very helpful indeed for some skiers.

The bindings, (which hold the boot to the ski) must be good ones and must have their tension checked frequently. This is very important as the binding must be individually adjusted for the particular skier so that it releases when the skier falls awkwardly. Care must also be taken when putting a boot into the binding to remove any lumps of snow or ice which tend to adhere to the sole of the boot, as they will prevent the binding from fitting properly. Most modern bindings are of the 'step in' type, where the foot can be pushed into the binding which then clicks into place. Some disabled people may, however, need someone to push their foot into the binding as the resistance is quite strong. This type of binding has two small prongs which anchor the ski to the snow while there is no boot in it, so that the ski cannot take off down the slope on its own if the boot comes out.

Some handicapped people will be helped by the use of outriggers rather than ski sticks. These vary slightly in design, especially those used by amputees, but are basically an elbow crutch with a short ski attached to the bottom. Some outriggers have a kind of metal claw at the back which can act as a brake. Some outriggers are rigid, whilst others have a little give through a piece of strong rubber into which the crutch is

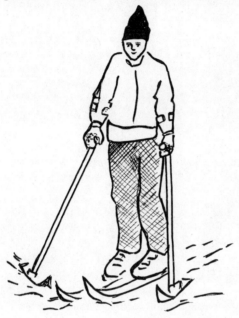

Outriggers help with balance on the snow

mounted at the join with the ski. New ideas are always being tried in the design of outriggers and different people will find slightly different adjustments will suit them best. The elbow crutch is adjustable, which means skiers of different heights can use the same pair. Outriggers are a marvellous invention which enable many people to enjoy skiing who could not otherwise manage. Their main disadvantages is that they tend to be very heavy, which can be quite a strain on the arms. People with various disabilities may benefit from using outriggers. People with some paralysis of one side of the body and who may only be able to use one arm, often find one outrigger helps greatly as it offsets the weakness in one leg. Amputees use two outriggers and many people with problems of balance or weakness of one or both legs will also be helped by their use.

Another very useful piece of equipment is the pole. This is a fairly long pole which is held at each end by an experienced skier and the disabled person holds the pole in the middle instead of using sticks or outriggers. This is used a lot in teaching blind people to ski. It is also very helpful with those who are quite severely handicapped, as it gives them a chance

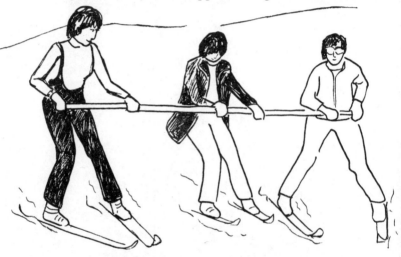

Learning to ski with the aid of a pole

to get used to the feeling of movement in an upright position which they may never otherwise have experienced. It also allows the skier to adjust to the feel of the skis on his feet and their gliding motion. It is important that the people at either end are fairly competent skiers and preferably not too dissimilar in height.

The 'steer ski' is another useful piece of equipment. This looks rather like a child's scooter but with a short ski instead of wheels on the bottom. It is very helpful for someone who has not got very good balance and finds it easier to lean forward and hold on to the 'handlebars' than to manage ski sticks or

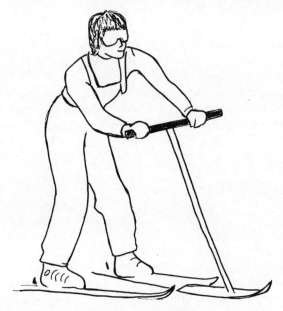

Using a steer ski

outriggers, at least in the early stages of learning to ski.

Other aids used to help blind skiers may include a whistle blown by a guide who skis in front of him. A competent guide is invaluable and may call out directions to the skier using an imaginary clock face to indicate the degree of turn required in either direction. For example a turn to the right would be indicated by the numbers 1 to 5 and to the left by 11 to 7. Using this method it is preferable for the instructor to ski behind the learner in order to judge the terrain from the skier's position. For a partially sighted skier it is best for the guide to ski in front. Ski sticks are very important to a blind skier for balance, help in turning, to push himself and to help judge the steepness of the slope. A ski stick may also be used to hold while the instructor guides him over a flat area or gentle slope. The long pole mentioned above, held by two sighted skiers, is of more use for a steeper slope.

Other methods used for blind skiers include holding on to the instructor's waist from behind, or with a beginner skiing backwards holding the learner's ski tips. These latter methods are also sometimes very useful in teaching a physically handicapped skier. Both methods help to build up the confidence of someone not used to moving on skis.

How to get up the slope

Getting back up the slope easily is very important to the downhill skier. In contrast to the cross country skier who will be happy to walk up a slope, the downhill skier will not want to do so. It takes a long time, is very hard work, and rigid downhill bindings and boots are not designed for easy climbing of slopes.

For this reason a variety of aids have been devised including ski tows of various kinds, chair lifts, cable cars, mountain railways and variations of these. Not all these types of lift are equally suitable for all disabled people. Cable cars and mountain railways can probably be used by most disabled skiers, if necessary with some assistance. Chair lifts may be very difficult to use and are not suitable for most people with epilepsy. The excitement and sensation of swinging out over space can easily trigger a fit which could be highly dangerous. Also some people with cerebral palsy may find that swinging in space causes their legs to go into spasm which may be painful and difficult to control. However, chair lifts may be used by some disabled people, including the blind, and can be managed by someone with two outriggers provided there is a strong assistant. It can also be helpful if the lift attendant will slow the lift down as the disabled skier gets on and off.

Ski tows may be fitted either with a cross bar which two people use together, with the bar behind them (it does help if the two people are roughly the same height!), or the 'poma' type popular in Italy, which has a plastic disc which is put between one's legs and pulls from behind. These tows require quite a bit of strength and dexterity to use but many disabled people do learn to manage them either by themselves or with help from a strong assistant.

Another type of tow is the rope tow. This is a length of rope which moves in a continuous round and is powered by a motor. The skier holds the rope and is pulled to the top of the slope. As may be imagined it is quite hard on the hands, and leather gloves or gardening gloves are required as the rope will very quickly ruin vinyl ski gloves. A rope tow is quite difficult to use; again, many disabled people learn to manage on their own, but the more severely disabled will probably require assistance. A strong helper stands behind the skier and pulls them both up on the tow. Skiers using ordinary sticks can usually tuck these under their arms, but someone with outriggers may need a helper to carry these up for him. As one young disabled skier summed up skiing: 'It's magic!'

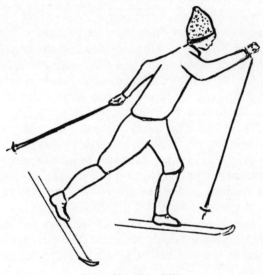

Nordic skiing

Cross country skiing
Another type of skiing is Nordic skiing (cross country) which is also called 'langlauf'. This consists of skiing along tracks which go both up and down hill – usually not too steeply! The movement is a rhythmic gliding which is a kind of cross between walking and running. The equipment used is slightly different from downhill equipment. The skis are narrower and longer, and may have pieces of fur or 'fish scale' markings on the sole to help prevent the ski slipping backwards on an incline. These make a curious swishing sound when going downhill. The bindings are very simple and are designed to

hold the boot only at the toe. The boots themselves are very light and flexible and more like a training shoe than a ski boot. They have a protruding welt at the toe which the binding grips. The object is to hold the foot firmly but leave the heel free to rise off the ski and the foot to bend. The ski sticks tend to be slightly longer than for downhill.

The clothing worn need not be as warm as for downhill skiing, as someone cross country skiing generates quite a bit of heat! Knickerbockers are often worn in preference to trousers as they leave the lower leg free.

Nordic skiing is becoming increasingly popular. It is a very pleasant sport and many people enjoy getting away from the crowded pistes and the queues for lifts. Many trails go through wooded country and may be very beautiful. Unfortunately it is not suitable for all disabled skiers as a fair degree of co-ordination is required, along with quite strong legs and the ability to raise the heel of the foot and bend the sole. However, some disabled people will certainly enjoy cross country skiing, and blind people, some mentally handicapped and the less severely physically disabled will probably be able to participate. Blind skiers can participate by feeling two parallel tracks made by a machine (or by following another skier's tracks) and will usually need a guide calling out directions about the slope, obstructions and so on. One blind skier has even participated in a 'ski-shooting' race in which he had to ski a certain distance and then shoot at a target before skiing a further distance.

Most resorts which offer cross country skiing will have a variety of trails of different lengths. Some of these will run through villages. This makes a very pleasant run, as one can ski some distance then stop for a drink, then ski on to the next village!

Other winter sports

Tobogganning: this is a sport that many quite severely handicapped people can enjoy. The main problem is getting back up the slope. If the handicapped person can walk up there is no problem; if, however, he cannot do so then it may need quite a strong person to pull him up! Ideally a ski lift could be used, but most ski resorts do not like people tobogganning on the ski runs, so unless there is another run not used by skiers this may not be possible.

Toboggans may be the traditional wooden type which can be used solo or with a helper. The modern plastic toboggans are also good fun to use and have the advantage that they can be steered (at least to some extent) by two brake levers, one at each side.

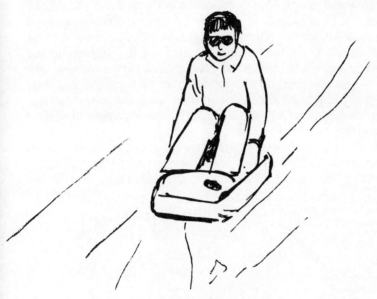

Toboggans are fun

Ski bobbing: a ski bob looks slightly like a bicycle with short skis instead of wheels. The rider sits on a saddle and holds on to the handlebars. On his feet he wears ski boots with a very short ski attached by a simple binding. These allow extra control and braking power. Ski bobs are rather clumsy to take on ski lifts, but can be managed on most types of tow, chairlift, cable car and so on, if necessary with assistance.

Ski bobbing is a very enjoyable sport and gives a satisfying feeling of speed and skill in manoeuvring. The Uphill Ski Club introduced ski bobbing to their holiday in St Johann in 1982 with great success. Handicapped people who enjoy skiing but who perhaps feel that they have stopped progressing may find that ski bobbing provides a stimulating new challenge, which can be very successfully mastered. People who have not skied may also of course enjoy ski bobbing and may find it a very pleasant introduction to winter sports.

Winter sports worldwide

Britain is not the only country to have developed winter sports for disabled people. Many countries in Europe and the United States of America have various schemes in operation. For example in Norway there is a hotel which specialises in cross country skiing in winter and orienteering in summer, which takes groups of handicapped visitors from various institutions in Norway. Most of the visitors are both physically and mentally handicapped. Some of them go cross country skiing and the more severely handicapped are pulled about in sledges or Norwegian 'pulks'.

In the United States of America a variety of winter sports have been developed for both the physically and mentally handicapped. Some of these are similar sports to those being

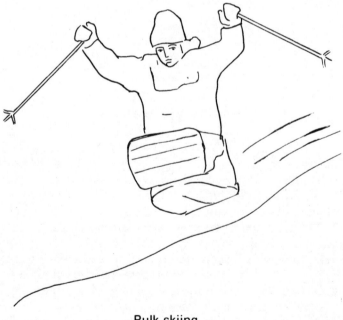

Pulk skiing

developed in Europe, such as downhill and cross country skiing, but others are only possible in areas with more snow and ice, such as ice fishing. Pulk skiing and sledding are new and interesting sports which could be developed in areas in Europe where there is skiing. Originating in Norway, pulks were used for over 100 years to carry cargo, while the Laplanders skiied beside them.

Pulks are a form of sled and the modern ones are usually made of fibre-glass. They are flat bottomed but the length and width vary with the purpose they are used for. Some sleds have been developed with metal edges on the bottom to allow more control. A severely disabled person, or a child, can be pulled in a pulk sled by someone wearing cross country skis, by means of a harness and two poles on the sled. Dog sledding can also be done by people too severely handicapped to push themselves; the dogs being attached to the pulk by a harness. Those whose arms are strong enough can propel the pulk themselves by using poles.

Ice sledding is similar to pulk skiing and was also developed in Norway. In the late 19th century the Norwegian fishermen

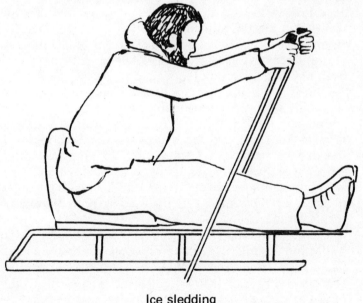

Ice sledding

used long wooden sleds to transport themselves across the ice to their winter fishing grounds and to carry their catch home. Ice sleds have blades on the bottom and can also be propelled by the use of poles. Ice sleds are used in Norway, Canada and in the United States for speed skating and a game similar to ice hockey.

Many of the special summer camps in America are able to operate exciting winter programmes for many handicapped people based on a wide range of snow and ice activities. One such camp provides winter adventure in the northern districts of Minnesota in the mid-west United States of America. The land of 10,000 lakes finds six months of the year with a three foot layer of solid blue ice covering the large expanses of freshwater. Minnesota, some have said, may not be the end of the world – 'but you can see it from there!' But that very same hard winter has enabled many local handicapped residents to participate in activities otherwise impossible. Dick Endres, the founder and director of Camp Confidence, writes:

Camp Confidence, in Brainerd, Minnesota, has proven itelf as a pioneer in the field of year-round camping and outdoor education with the handicapped – primarily mentally retarded. Camp Confidence, developed on 140 acres of virgin land and possessing over half a mile of lakeshore on beautiful Sylvan Lake, is unique and different in many ways from any other camp in the United States.

Camp Confidence operates twelve months a year, free of charge to mentally retarded citizens of all ages.

Campers are not sent to Camp Confidence – they are brought to camp by the agency or family booking in reservations with us. Agency staff or family members remain with their campers and serve as 'counsellors'. There is no central dining hall at Camp Confidence, nor is one ever planned. All the campers are involved in the preparation of their own meals.

The heart of Camp Confidence is the programme staff of professional outdoor education specialists who have modi-fied a wide variety of activities and assist the campers and accompanying staff in the implementation of them. Emphasis at Camp Confidence is upon 'learning by doing'; to develop both a feeling of self-confidence through accomplishment and a consideration of one's fellow man. I have observed many times the frustration experienced by the mentally retarded. Their entire life has been one of failure. They hesitate very much in trying anything new and 'failing again'. It is vital to note here the importance of a positive staff attitude. We at Camp Confidence believe the mentally retarded should have the opportunity to experience life to the full. There are so many things we can do *with* them, not *for* them . . . Many things they themselves do not realize they can do – but are great confidence builders and develop a feeling of self worth within the individual.

The most popular winter sport at Camp Confidence is our tubing run. This is a 300 foot 'S'-curved trail, or trough, cut into one of our many hills. It has natural embankments four to eight feet high on both sides of the run. A minimum of six inches of snow is all that is necessary to make this run operable. Truck innertubes are obtained and the long curved valve stem is replaced with a short stubby one – for safety reasons. A few relatively slow initial rides down the run quickly pack the snow into a firm base. Subsequent riders gain additional speed and flare out in following the natural contour of the curves to pack the restraining banks. It is extremely important to have adequate restraining banks as it is impossible to actually 'steer' the innertube down the hard packed 'S'-curved surface. Properly constructed, the tubing run is a safe, exciting, and popular activity for all. Some campers ride the tubes down lying on their backs. Others lie on their chests and hips. The innertubes are soft and 'bouncy', this makes it safe to send four or five riders down at one time. They act somewhat like bumper cars, rebounding off one another.

We have also lined up ten or more innertubes in sequence with all riders on their backs and holding on to the feet of the person behind them – who places their feet under the armpits of the person ahead. This ride produces a 'snakey' train effect with a maximum of 'hoots and hollers'. One of our campers, whom I'll call Jack, comes to camp several times a year from Western Minnesota. Jack is confined to a wheelchair, as are many of our users. Jack was fascinated with watching his friends zoom down the tubing run; he was given a ride up the hill on an all-terrain vehicle and helped onto a tube. As he put it afterwards: 'Maybe I can't walk, but I can sure ride!'

Snow skiing is a universally popular winter sport. Camp Confidence has developed a very successful programme – both cross country and downhill, or alpine, skiing. Most campers start with the less frightening cross country activity. Never having had skis on their feet before, they can gain the feeling of 'the boards' and of sliding them along a relatively flat pre-laid trail with an almost instant feeling of accomplishment. Two years ago we added a new dimension to this programme – cross country skiing with the mentally retarded, blind, campers. Our staff developed it's own technique by standing in front of the blind skier and straddling his skis. The blind skier would place his hands on the staff's elbows. We then talked the camper through the gliding experience. On occasion this initial instruction was followed with a request from the blind skier: 'Let me try it alone.' What a thrill for us when the skier shrieked: 'I'm doing it, I'm doing it!'

Downhill, or alpine, skiing with the mentally retarded may be viewed by some as too risky. Again, a positive staff attitude is most important. If you believe 'they can't do this', you're probably right – they won't! The Camp Confidence downhill skiing programme is an excellent example of doing things with the mentally retarded which they do not realize they can do. It is a great confidence builder through personal achievement.

We have cleared our own skiing hill and have installed a rope tow – through community help. In 1973 we introduced the graduated length method (GLM) of skiing. This method employs the use of short skis, 100 centimetres long. These 'shorty' skis provide much better control and ability to make turns. They also make it much easier to right oneself after falling. Our hill is designed to enable skiers to begin their descent at various levels – from the very gradual to the more inclined. Proper foot gear and quick release binding are essential. Donated equipment was obtained by solicitation from area ski shops.

When the snow is twelve inches or more in depth the snowshoes come out. These elongated 'tennis racquets' are clumsy and awkward to walk on. They are fascinating, however, as the campers experience walking on top of the snow. They are also useful in developing confidence and co-ordination. Snowshoes provide the opportunity to explore the depth of the woods and observe many of nature's winter creatures. One of our campers best described snowshoeing to me; he said: 'It's like trying to walk after you wet your pants!'

Ice fishing is another fascinating Minnesota winter sport. When there are six inches or more of solid blue ice, fish houses are pushed out onto the lake. Fish houses are small shanties of various shapes and decor. On our larger Minnesota lakes you will see literally thousands of fish houses merging into actual villages on the ice. Camp Confidence fish houses are eight feet square and seven feet high. The wooden floor is carpeted and the walls and ceiling are insulated with styrofoam. A twelve-inch square hole is located in each corner of the floor. Small windows in the walls provide daytime lighting. The fish house is equipped with a small stove – either wood burning or propane. The fish house is located on a likely spot, elevated off the ice on blocks, and banked up with snow. Holes are then chipped or augered in the ice exposed in the four corners. This is no small chore when the ice reaches three foot thick proportions.

Fishing lines are rigged with hook, sinker and float bobber. Excess line is kept on a wooden reel attached to the wall above each hole. Minnows of various sizes are used for bait. The bait is lowered to various depths, but usually approximately 12 inches off the bottom, and the bobber set.

The small stove warms the interior of the fish house very quickly. Jackets are removed and one can sit in relative comfort in shirtsleeves – although the temperature outside may be 30 degrees F below zero! This could appear to be a ridiculous amount of effort – just to catch a fish. True, but like most activities, the preparation is often as enjoyable as the activity itself.

Other popular ice sports at Camp Confidence are ice

skating and broomball. Many of our campers have never had skates on their feet. Just to stand on them is difficult. A simple device to assist them is a straight-back kitchen chair. The skater can stand behind the chair, hold on to the top of it and slowly push it along the ice. Broomball is an excellent activity which can be modified in many ways. It is a take-off from ice hockey. Rig up two make-shift goals, give everyone an old broom, and toss a soccer ball out onto the ice. Players swat the ball along with their brooms and chase it along the ice. We do not use ice skates for broomball, although they can be used for higher functioning individuals. By eliminating ice skates, many more campers can participate.

Another exhilarating experience on the ice is the use of Swedish kick sleds. They are an Alaskan type of dog sled with narrow steel runners. We use these with our physically handicapped campers and refer to them as our winter wheelchairs.

Snowmobiling has grown into a very popular sport in Minnesota. Snowmobiles are a part of our winter programme at Camp Confidence. They are used primarily as a work or transportation vehicle, again for our physically handicapped campers . . . ie. for transporting wheelchair campers to the fish house. Individual campers do not operate these high powered machines – for two reasons: for reasons of safety and because we wish our users to participate in activities which demand their physical involvement as much as possible – *doing it under their own power* and not relying upon a machine.

Outdoor cooking is a great camping experience, but certainly not during the winter. My immediate response again: 'Why not!' Many Camp Confidence camping groups enjoy cooking over an open wood fire during mild winter days. Those hamburgers, hot dogs, beans, etc., really taste fantastic following a two hour cross country trek on the 'back 80.' Please let it be noted that we do not throw caution to the winds and demand that our campers survive under extreme conditions. The use of proper clothing, including the layer system, is taught. Staff are constantly checking for frostbite. The wind chill factor is probably the most vital factor to be aware of. Many activities can be enjoyed in close to zero F temperatures providing there is no wind. On the other hand, 20 degrees above zero with a 15 mile an hour wind can be very cutting and bitterly cold to exposed skin areas.

Yes, camping can be a most enjoyable and educational experience – on a year-round basis; an experience not reserved only for the hale and hardy – but also for the handicapped. We are proving it at Camp Confidence in Brainerd, Minnesota.

How to go about trying winter sports

Any handicapped person who wishes to try a winter sports holiday would be well advised to contact one of the following organisations. The Uphill Ski Club provides recreational skiing and ski bobbing for people with most types of physical or slight mental handicap. The British Ski Club for the Disabled specialises in teaching blind skiers and amputees and also organises participation in competitive events for the Winter Olympics for the Disabled.

Both organisations are charities relying on donations and voluntary help. Both are very willing to help any disabled person who wishes to try winter sports. There are a wide range of aids which may need to be adapted to suit the individual. Many disabled people get much pleasure out of various winter sports, and the equipment which has been developed over the years enables many to participate who would not otherwise be able.

So if you are looking for a new interest or challenge in adventure, it may be waiting for you on snow-covered mountain slopes. The thrill of the down-hill ski course, a journey across country through spruce and fir woods or a gentle toboggan ride; the opportunities are there. Never again need the handicapped person be just another spectator.

Appendices

I Further Reading

Introduction

An Introduction to Adventure: a sequential approach to challenging activities with persons who are disabled, C.Roland and M.Havens, Vinland National Center, 1981 (available from Vinland Center, Loretto, Minnesota 55357, USA.)

Directory of centres for outdoor studies in England and Wales, Council for Environmental Education, 1981

Games, Sports and Exercises for the physically handicapped, R.Adams *et al*, Lea and Febiger (Philadelphia), 1975, (available from Henry Kimpton, 205 Great Portland Street, London W1).

Holidays for the physically handicapped, Royal Association for Disability and Rehabilitation, 1979

Give us the chance: sport and physical recreation with mentally handicapped people, Disabled Living Foundation, 1981

In Touch, M.Ford & T.Heshel, BBC Publications, 1977

Informal Countryside Recreation for Disabled People (Advisory Series No.15), The Countryside Commission, 1981

Outdoor Opportunities for People with Mental Handicap, The Sports Council UK, 1983

Out of Doors with Handicapped People, M.Cotton, Souvenir Press, 1981.

Outdoor Pursuits for Disabled People, N.Croucher, Woodhead-Faulkner (for the Disabled Living Foundation), 1981

The Bradford Papers (Proceedings from the Annual Institute on Innovations in Camping and Outdoor Education with Persons who are Disabled), (vols.I and II). ed G.Robb, Bradford Woods (University of Indiana), 1981–1982

The Duke of Edinburgh's Award: Handbook and *Guide for the Handicapped*, 1980

Chapter 1:   In the Water
Life Saving, Royal LifeSaving Association, London, 1975
Swimming for the Disabled, Association of Swimming Therapy,
EP Publishing Ltd., 1981
The Diving Manual, British Sub-Aqua Club, 1979
The Teaching of Swimming, Amateur Swimming Association,
Loughborough, 1974

Chapter 2:   Life Afloat
Sailing from Start to Finish, Y.Pinaud, Adlard Coles, 1975
Starting Sailing, J.Moore & A.Turvey, David & Charles, 1974
The Sailing Instructor's Guide, W.B.Keeble & D.W.Cobden,
Kandy, 1971
The Sailing Manual, B.Bond, Pelham Books, London, 1973
The Yachtsman's Weather Map, F.Singleton & K.Best, RYA,
1977
They said we couldn't do it, RYA Seamanship Foundation, 1981
This is Racing, R.Creagh-Osborne, Nautical, 1977
Water Sports for the Disabled, RYA Seamanship Foundation,
(revised ed.), 1983

Chapter 3:   Just Paddling About
Canoeing Handbook, British Canoe Union
'Disabled Update', in *Canoe Focus*, British Canoe Union,
Spring 1983
Know the Game: Canoeing, EP Publications Ltd.
Puffin Adventure Sports: Canoeing, P.Little & D.English,
Puffin Books, 1981
The Starting Series: Canoeing, A.Williams & D.Piercey, Barrie
& Jenkins, 1980

Chapter 4:   At the Water's Edge
Fishing Facilities for Disabled in Scotland, Committee for
promotion of angling for disabled, 1982
Guide to Fishing Facilities for the Disabled Angler, National
Anglers Council, 1977
Guide to Outdoor Activities for the handicapped, Country
Landowners' Association Charitable Trust, 1983
Teach Yourself Fishing, Royal National Institute for the Blind,
(available from RNIB as 2 vols. in braille)

Chapter 5: In the saddle
Introduction to Riding for the Disabled, G.Peacock & S. Saywell, Riding for the Disabled Association
Riding for the Disabled Association Handbook, RDA

Chapter 6: Out on the Hills
Adventure walking for young people, F.Duerden, Kaye & Ward, 1980
EP Sport Orienteering, M.Henley, EP Publishing, 1976
Lost Canals of England and Wales, R.Russell, David & Charles
Orienteering, J.Disley, Faber, 1978
Tackle Rambling, A.Mattingly, Stanley Paul, 1981
The Shell Book of Inland Waterways, H.McKnight, David & Charles
Walking in the countryside, D.Sharp, David & Charles, 1978

Chapter 7: Going to Camp
Bernese Alps Expedition, The Spastics Society, 1977
Better camping, A. Ryalls & R. Marchant, Kaye & Ward, 1973
Camping, R.Jeffries & P.Moynihan, MacDonald, 1982
Churchtown Farm Hebrides Expedition, The Spastics Society, 1981
Enjoy Camping, Scout Association, 1973
EP Sport Backpacking, D.Robinson, EP Publishing, 1981
The Backpacker's Handbook, D.Booth, Letts, 1975
The Duke of Edinburgh's Award – Expedition Guide, ed. R.Ransom,. 1981
The Expedition Handbook, ed.T.Land, Butterworths, 1978
The Usborne Outdoor Book, Usborne, 1979

Chapter 8: Reaching High and Low
Adventure Education and Outdoor Pursuits, C.J.Mortlock, Charlotte Mason College of Education, Ambleside
Artificial Climbing Walls, K.Meldrum, Pelham Books
EP Sport Rock Climbing, P.Livesey, EP Publishing, 1978
High Hopes, N.Croucher, Hodder & Stoughton, 1976
Improvised techniques in Mountain Rescue, W.March, Plas y Brenin.
Know the Game: Potholing and Caving, EP Publishing Ltd.

Manual of Caving Techniques, ed. Cullingford, Routledge & Kegan Paul, 1979

Mountain and Cave Rescue, Mountain Rescue Committee, Sports Council

Modern Snow and Ice Techniques, W.March, Plas y Brenin

Mountain Leadership Handbook, E. Langmuir, Scottish Sports Council, Edinburgh

Mountaineering, A.Blackshaw, Penguin

Safety in Outdoor Pursuits, HMSO

The Hard Years, J. Brown, Gollance

The Starting Series: Rock Climbing, A.Clarke, Barrie & Jenkins

Chapter 9: Winter Sports

Disabled Teaching Methods M.Hammond, British Ski Club for the Disabled (BSCD)

Pulk skiing and ice sledding for persons with mobility impairments, D.Abell & L.Orr, Vinland National Center, Minnesota, 1981

Skiing as a means of therapy for physically handicapped children, L.Williams, (available from BSCD), 1973

Where there's a Will, M.Brace, Souvenir Press, 1980

II   Films

Able to Fish – 1 Coarse Angling 2 Game Fishing 3 Sea Fishing
Give us the Chance (mixed sport and recreation for mentally handicapped people)
Not Just a Spectator (mixed sport and recreation for disabled people)
Riding for the Disabled (this and the following two films are based on the Riding for the Disabled Association)
Riding towards Freedom
The Right to Choose
Water Free (presented by the Association of Swimming Therapy)

For hire and purchase of all of these films apply in writing to: Town and Country Productions Ltd., 21, Cheyne Row, Chelsea, London SW3 5HP

Cold Water can kill
Lifejackets and personal buoyancy aids
On the water, in the water
Water safety code

Available from: The Royal Society for the Prevention of Accidents, Cannon House, The Priory, Queensway, Birmingham B4 6BS

An adventure playground for the handicapped

Available from: The Central Film Library, Government Building, Bromyard Ave., Acton, London W3 7JB

III   Useful Addresses

Introduction
Bradford Woods Outdoor Education Center, c/o Dr Gary Robb, University of Indiana, Martinsville, Indiana, USA.
British Sports Association for the Disabled, Sir Ludwig Guttman Sports Centre, Harvey Road, Aylesbury, Bucks. HP21 8PP.
Calvert Trust Adventure Centre, Old Windebrow, Keswick, Cumbria CA12 4NT.
Calvert Trust Adventure Centre, Keilder Forest, Northumberland.
Churchtown Farm Field Studies Centre, Lanlivery, Bodmin, Cornwall.
Country Landowners' Association Charitable Trust, Bohune Common House, Woodborough, Pewsey, Wilts.
Disabled Living Foundation, 346 Kensington High Street, London W14 8NS.
English Tourist Board, 4 Grosvenor Gardens, London SW1W ODU.
Forestry Commission, 231 Corstorphine Road, Edinburgh EH12 7AT.
Handicapped Adventure Playground Association, Fulham Palace, Bishops Avenue, London SW6.
Institute of Park and Recreation Administration, Lower Basildon, Reading, Berks. RG8 9NE.
Low Mill Youth Centre, Askrigg, Wensleydale, N.Yorkshire.
National Association for Outdoor Education, Beverley Park Centre (Outdoor Pursuits), Pateley Bridge, Nr. Harrogate, N.Yorks.
National Federation of Gateway Clubs, 117–23 Golden Lane, London EC1Y 0RT.
National PHAB, 42 Devonshire Street, London W1N 1LN.
Outward Bound Trust, Avon House, 360 Oxford Street, London W1.
Royal Association for Disability and Rehabilitation, 25 Mortimer Street, London W1N 8AB.
Scottish Sports Association for the Disabled, Secretary: R.C.Brickley, Fife Institute of Physical Education, Viewfield Road, Glenrothes, Fife, KY6 2RA.

Scottish Sports Council, 1 St Colme Street, Edinburgh EH3 6AA.

Scottish Tourist Board, 23 Ravelston Terrace, Edinburgh 4.

Sports Club for the Blind, Secretary: Miss E.Wright, Flat 4, 27 Underhill Road, Dulwich, London SE22.

The Countryside Commission, John Dower House, Crescent Place, Cheltenham, Glos. GL50 3RA.

The Countryside Commission for Scotland, Battleby, Redgorton, Perth PH1 3EW.

The Nature Conservancy Council, 19–20 Belgrave Square, London SW1X 8PY.

The National Trust, 42 Queen Anne's Gate, London SW1.

The Northern Ireland Information Service for the Disabled, 2 Annadale Avenue, Belfast BT7 3JH.

The SHARE Centre, Smith's Strand, Upper Lough Erne, Shanaghy, Nr.Lisnaskea, Co.Fermanagh, N.Ireland.

The Sports Council, 16 Upper Woburn Place, London WC1H OQP.

The Wales Council for the Disabled, Crescent Road, Caerphilly, Mid Glamorgan, CF8 1XL.

United Kingdom Sports Association for People with Mental Handicap, c/o The Sports Council, 16 Upper Woburn Place, London WC1H 0QP.

Vinland National Center, 3675 Ihduhapi Road, PO Box 308, Loretto, Minnesota, 55357, USA

Wales Sports Association for the Disabled, c/o Sports Council for Wales, National Sports Centre for Wales, Sophia Gardens, Cardiff CF1 9SW.

Wales Tourist Board, Welcome House, Llandaff, Cardiff.

Winged Fellowship Trust (Holidays for the Disabled), 64–66 Oxford Street, London W1N 9FF.

Chapter 1: In the Water

Amateur Swimming Association, Harold Fern House, Derby Square, Loughborough, Leics. LE11 0AL.

Association of Swimming Therapy, 1 Buchan Grove, Crewe, Cheshire.

British Sub-Aqua Club, 70 Brompton Road, London SW3 1HA.

National Association of Swimming Clubs for the Handicapped, 63 Dunvegan Road, Eltham, London SE9.

National Co-ordinating Committee on Swimming for the Disabled, Swimming Teachers' Association, 1 Birmingham Road, West Bromwich, West Midlands BT1 4JQ.

The Royal Life Saving Society, Desborough House, 14 Devonshire Street, London W1N 2AT.

Swimming Teachers' Association, 1 Birmingham Road, West Bromwich, West Midlands BT1 4JQ.

Chapter 2: Life Afloat

Central Council for the Disabled, 34 Eccleston Square, London SW1V 1PE.

Inland Waterways Association, 114 Regents Park Road, London NW1 8UQ.

National School Sailing Association, c/o D.Sykes, 14 Chambrai Close, Appleford, Abingdon, Oxfordshire OX14 4NT.

Peter le Marchant Trust, c/o Colston Bassett House, Colston Bassett, Nottingham NG12 3FE.

Royal Yachting Association and *RYA Seamanship Foundation*, Victoria Way, Woking, Surrey GU21 1EQ.

Thames Cruises, c/o Wansborough Manor, Guildford GU3 2JR.

The Jubilee Sailing Trust, Beauvoir Lodge, Effingham Lane, Copthorne, Sussex.

Water Space Amenity Commission, 1 Queen Anne's Gate, London SW1H 9BT.

Water Sports Division, British Sports Association for the Disabled, 29 Ironlatch Avenue, St Leonards-on-Sea, E Sussex TN38 9JF.

Chapter 3: Just Paddling About

The British Canoe Union, Flexel House, 45–7 High Street, Addlestone, Weybridge, Surrey KT15 1JV.

The Canoe Camping Club, 9 Glebe Road, Sandy, Beds. SG19 1LS.

Chapter 4: At the Water's Edge

Committee for the Promotion of Angling for the Disabled, (Scotland), Mrs M.Taylor, 18–19 Claremont Crescent, Edinburgh.

National Anglers' Council, Committee for Disabled Anglers, Cowgate, Peterborough.

National Federation of Anglers, Halliday House, 2 Wilson Street, Derby DE1 1PG.

National Federation of Sea Anglers, 26 Downsview Crescent, Uckfield, Sussex TN22 1UB.

Regional Water Authorities:

Anglia Diploma House, Grammar School Walk, Huntingdon PE18 6NZ.

Northumbria Northumbria House, Regent Centre, Gosforth, Newcastle-upon-Tyne.

North West Dawson House, Great Sankey, Warrington WA5 3LW.

Severn Trent Abelson House, 2297 Coventry Road, Sheldon, Birmingham.

South West 3–5 Barnfield Road, Exeter EX1 1RE.

Southern Guildbourne House, Worthing, Sussex BN11 1LD.

Thames New River Head, Rosebery Avenue, London EC1R 4TP.

Wessex Techno House, Redcliffe Way, Bristol BS1 6NY.

Yorkshire West Riding House, 67 Albion Street, Leeds LS1 5AA.

Salmon and Trout Association, Fishmongers' Hall, London EC4R 9EL.

Water Sports Division, British Sports Association for the Disabled, 29 Ironlatch Avenue, St Leonards-on-Sea, East Sussex YN38 9JE.

Chapter 5: In the Saddle

British Horse Society, National Equestrian Centre, Stoneleigh, Kenilworth, Warks. CV8 2LR.

Diamond Riding Centre for the Handicapped, Carshalton, Surrey.

English Riding Holiday and Trekking Association, National Equestrian Centre, Stoneleigh, Kenilworth, Warks. CV8 2LR.

Riding for the Disabled Association, Avenue 'R', National Agricultural Centre, Stoneleigh, Kenilworth, Warks. CV8 2LY.

The Pony Club, National Equestrian Centre, Stoneleigh, Kenilworth, Warks. CV8 2LR.

Chapter 6: Out on the Hills
British Orienteering Federation, Lea Green, Nr. Matlock, Derby DE4 5GJ.
Cyclists' Touring Club, Cotterell House, 69 Meadrow, Godalming, Surrey GU7 7HS.
Ramblers' Association, Crawford Mews, York Street, London W1H 1PT.
Silva Compasses (London) Ltd., 76 Broad Street, Teddington TW11 8QT.
The Scottish Youth Hostels Association, 7 Glebe Crescent, Stirling FK8 2JA.
The Youth Hostels Association, Trevelyan House, St Stephen's Hill, St Albans, Herts.

Chapter 7: Going to Camp
Camping Club of Great Britain and Ireland, 11 Lower Grosvenor Place, London SW1W 0EY.
The Duke of Edinburgh's Award Scheme, 5 Prince of Wales Terrace, London W8 5PG.
The Girl Guides Association, 17 Buckingham Palace Road, London SW1 0PT.
The Scout Association, Baden Powell House, Queens Gate, London SW7
The Youth Camping Association of Great Britain and Ireland, 91 Hurst Drive, Waltham Cross, Herts.
Woodlarks Camp, Tilford Road, Farnham, Surrey.

Chapter 8: Reaching High and Low
British Mountaineering Council, Crawford House, Booth Street East, Manchester M13 9RZ.
Deaf Mountaineering Club, c/o British Deaf Association, 38 Victoria Place, Carlisle CA1 1HU.
Federation of Mountaineering Clubs, Ireland Secretary: Miss P.Hamilton, 27 Landseer Street, Belfast 9.
Grampian Speleological Group, Secretary: Mr.A.Jeffreys, 8 Scone Gardens, Edinburgh EH8 7DQ.
Irish Caving Club, Secretary: Mr.M.Rendle, 10 Morham Street, Belfast 7.
Mountain Rescue Committee, 9 Milldale Avenue, Temple Meads, Buxton, Derbyshire SK17 9BE.

Mountaineering Council of Scotland, Secretary: Mr W.M.S. Myles, 59 Morningside Park, Edinburgh 9.
National Caving Association, Secretary: Mr D.Judson, Bethnal Green, Calderbrook Road, Littleborough, Lancs.

Chapter 9: Winter Sports
British Ski Club for the Deaf, c/o British Deaf Association, 38 Victoria Place, Carlisle CA1 1HU.
British Ski Club for the Disabled, c/o Hubert Sturges, Corton House, Corton, Warminster, Wilts. BA12 0SZ.
Camp Confidence, c/o Dick Endres, Camp Confidence, PO Box 349, Brainerd, Minnesota 56401, USA.
National Ski Federation of Great Britain, 118 Eaton Square, London SW1W 9AF.
Ski-bob Association of Great Britain, Secretary: Mr A.E.Marsh, 34 Lavant Street, Petersfield, Hants.
The Uphill Ski Club, 12 Park Crescent, London W1N 4EQ.

*Note that many of the above addresses are those of the Secretary, and are often home addresses. Consequently it is possible that with change of officers of the organisation, many will not be correct, although the person contacted should be able to inform you of the most recent address.

Index